A Concise Guide to Clinical Trials

A Concise Guide to Clinical Trials

Second Edition

Allan Hackshaw

WILEY Blackwell

Registered Offices
John Wiley & Sons, Inc., 111 River Street, Hoboken, NJ 07030, USA
John Wiley & Sons Ltd, The Atrium, Southern Gate, Chichester, West Sussex, PO19 8SQ, UK

For details of our global editorial offices, customer services, and more information about Wiley products visit us at www.wiley.com.

Wiley also publishes its books in a variety of electronic formats and by print-on-demand. Some content that appears in standard print versions of this book may not be available in other formats.

Library of Congress Cataloging-in-Publication Data
Names: Hackshaw, Allan K., author.
Title: A concise guide to clinical trials / Dr Allan Hackshaw.
Description: Second edition. | Hoboken, NJ : Wiley-Blackwell 2024. |
  Includes bibliographical references and index.
Identifiers: LCCN 2023052502 (print) | LCCN 2023052503 (ebook) | ISBN
  9781119502807 (paperback) | ISBN 9781119502777 (adobe pdf) | ISBN
  9781119502760 (epub)
Subjects: MESH: Clinical Trials as Topic
Classification: LCC RM301.27 (print) | LCC RM301.27 (ebook) | NLM W
  20.55.C5 | DDC 615.5072/4–dc23/eng/20240105
LC record available at https://lccn.loc.gov/2023052502
LC ebook record available at https://lccn.loc.gov/2023052503

Cover Design: Wiley
Cover Image: © Ted Horowitz Photography/Getty Images

Set in 9.5/12pt Palatino by Straive, Pondicherry, India

Contents

Preface

Clinical trials are essential for evaluating ways of preventing, detecting or treating disorders, or preventing early death. They are central to the work of many research departments including those in universities, hospitals, governmental organisations and pharmaceutical/medical device companies.

Health professionals conduct their own trials or engage in trials by recruiting participants, and others are involved in decision-making for grant funding, drug/medical device approval or developing clinical guidelines. There also many trial managers and those who analyse trials (research staff, statisticians and co-ordinators). All need to understand how new interventions are evaluated for themselves, and especially to be able to explain the benefits and harms to patients or the public. This book provides an overview of the design, conduct and interpretation of trials. No prior knowledge is required.

This is a significantly revised second edition, in which many new items have been added, including modern phase I to III study designs, trial designs for licencing and market access, translational research and precision medicine (incorporating biomarkers), and indirect treatment comparisons and real-world data as supporting evidence. There is also greater clarification of non-inferiority trials, health-related quality of life and subgroup analyses. Many examples used throughout the book are based on medicinal products (drugs) as these represent a substantial number of trials in practice. However, their design and analysis features can easily be applied to other interventions, and specific aspects of these are provided in Chapter 8.

I have spent over 32 years designing, conducting, analysing and publishing numerous clinical studies for various disorders (prevention, screening and treatment), from prenatal to the elderly. The book contains many practical tips that are not readily available in the literature. Much of this book has been based on successful courses on clinical trials delivered to a wide range of people: undergraduates, postgraduates and clinical and non-clinical health professionals in many academic institutions and pharmaceutical companies. The topics raised by them and how they have been taught and discussed have influenced the presentation of many concepts throughout the book

The book should be an easy-to-read guide that can be used as an introduction to clinical trials and as a teaching aid. It also contains enough information for those who wish to know more about a topic, and as a helpful reference guide to those already working in clinical trials.

Allan Hackshaw
Professor of Epidemiology & Medical Statistics
Director of the Cancer Research UK & UCL Cancer Trials Centre,
University College London
(previously at the Wolfson Institute of Preventive Medicine,
Queen Mary University of London)

Foreword

No one would doubt the importance of clinical trials in the progress and practice of medicine today. They have developed enormously over the past 80 years and have made significant contributions to our knowledge about the efficacy of new treatments, particularly in quantifying the magnitude of their effects. Clinical trials have become highly sophisticated, in their design, conduct, statistical analysis and the processes required before new medicines can be legally sold. They have become expensive and require large teams of experts covering pharmacology, statistics, computing, health economics and epidemiology, to mention only a few. The systematic combination of the results from many trials to provide clearer results, in the form of meta-analyses, have themselves developed their own sophistication and importance.

In all this panoply of activity and complexity, it is easy to lose sight of the elements that form the basis of good science and practice in the conduct of clinical trials. Allan Hackshaw, in this book, achieves this with great skill. He informs the general reader of the essential elements of clinical trials: the different forms of trial design and analyses and how trials are conducted.

As well as dealing with scientific issues, this book is useful in describing the terminology and procedures used in connection with clinical trials, including explanations of phase I, II and III trials, and real-world data. The book outlines the regulations governing the conduct of clinical trials and those that relate to the approval of new medicines – an area that has become complicated.

This book educates the general medical and scientific reader on clinical trials without requiring detailed knowledge in any particular area. It provides an up-to-date overview of clinical trials with commendable clarity.

Professor Sir Nicholas Wald FRS
Formerly, Director, Wolfson Institute of Environmental & Preventive Medicine
Barts and The London School of Medicine & Dentistry

CHAPTER 1

Fundamental concepts

This chapter provides a summary of the main types of trials and their key design features. A checklist for critical appraisal of trial reports is on page 199, and a glossary of common abbreviations is on page 201.

1.1 What is a clinical trial?

The two distinct study designs used in health research are **observational** and **experimental**. Observational studies (usually cross-sectional, retrospective case-control or prospective cohort) do not intentionally involve intervening in the way individuals live their lives or how they are treated.[1] However, clinical trials (experimental) are specifically designed to intervene, and then evaluate health-related outcomes, with the following objectives:

- To diagnose or detect a disease
- To prevent a disease or early death (prolong life)
- To treat or cure an existing disorder, including reducing or managing symptoms
- To change behaviour or lifestyle habits, including reducing risk factors.

Countries (low, middle and high income areas) can successfully conduct clinical trials that reflect local health issues. The fundamental features of design and analysis are similar but the conduct and delivery will vary (especially how interventions are administered and how follow-up and outcome data are collected).

An intervention could be a single therapy involving a substance that is injected, infused, swallowed, inhaled or absorbed through the skin; medical device; surgical procedure; radiotherapy; behavioural or psychological therapy; something to improve health service delivery or promote health education; or an alternative or complementary therapy.

A new generation of **biological and targeted therapies** (small molecules, monoclonal antibodies, immunotherapies and genetic and cell therapies) has revolutionised the treatment of several disorders, in which the choice of a therapy is influenced by the presence (or absence) of a biomarker, genetic abnormality or imaging marker. There are also **vaccines** that can be used for disease prevention or to reduce the risk of disease progression.

A combination of interventions can be referred to as a **regimen**, such as chemotherapy and surgery in treating cancer.

Any drug or micronutrient that is examined in a clinical trial with the specific purpose of treating, preventing or diagnosing disease is usually referred to as an **Investigational Medicinal Product (IMP)** or **Investigational New Drug (IND)**.[#] Most clinical trial regulations cover studies using an IMP and several medical devices.

[#] IMP in the UK and European Union, and IND in the United States, Canada and Japan.

A Concise Guide to Clinical Trials, Second Edition. Allan Hackshaw.
© 2024 John Wiley & Sons Ltd. Published 2024 by John Wiley & Sons Ltd.

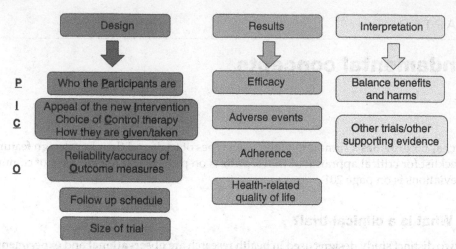

Figure 1.1 Overall view of trial design, types of results and interpretation. The acronym PICO (Participants/ Population, Intervention, Control and Outcome) focuses on the four key design elements that must always be clearly defined (examples of trials in later chapters use the PICO list). Translational research (bio- and imaging markers) can also be examined.

New drugs and some medical devices usually require a **licence** or **marketing authorisation** for human use from a national regulatory authority. They can then be made available to the target population after review by a **health technology assessment (HTA)** or **payer/reimbursement** organisation through a process referred to as **market access**.

Throughout this book, the terms **intervention**, **treatment** and **therapy** are used interchangeably. People who take part in a trial are referred to as **participants** if they are healthy individuals or **patients** if they are already ill with the disorder of interest.

Figure 1.1 is an overall view of trial design and types of results (covered in more detail in other chapters).

Patient and Public Involvement and Engagement (PPIE) is a key activity in which lay members (e.g. past patients, carers and members of the public) can help with trial design (e.g. agree that the new therapy is appealing), conduct (create the participant-facing information materials) and interpret trials in a way that can be easily understood.

Artificial intelligence is also expected to be used, for example in identifying eligible participants from electronic medical records and analysing clinical data and multiple biomarkers.

Decentralised trials may be increasingly used where many or all of the processes from participant selection and eligibility, allocation of treatments (usually licensed products already in use), through to data and outcome collection are done electronically including remote assessments of participants.

1.2 Early trials

James Lind, a Scottish naval physician, is regarded as conducting the first clinical trial.[2] During a sea voyage in 1747, he chose 12 sailors with *similarly* severe cases of scurvy and examined 6 treatments, each given to 2 sailors: cider, diluted sulphuric acid, vinegar, seawater, a mixture of foods including nutmeg and garlic, and oranges and lemons. These sailors were made to live in the *same* part of the ship and given the *same* basic diet. Lind understood the importance of standardising their living conditions to ensure that any change in their disease would unlikely be influenced by other factors. After about a week, both sailors given fruit had almost completely recovered unlike the other sailors. This dramatic effect led to the conclusion that eating fruit cured scurvy, without knowing that it was due to vitamin C.

Two important features of his trial were a **comparison** between two or more interventions and an attempt to ensure that the participants had **similar characteristics** (see confounding below). The requirement for these two features has not changed for more than 270 years, indicating how essential they are to evaluating interventions.

One key element missing from Lind's trial was the process of **randomisation**. The Medical Research Council trial of streptomycin and tuberculosis in 1948 is regarded as the first to use random allocation.[3]

1.3 Why clinical trials are needed

Statin therapy is effective in treating coronary heart disease. However, why do some patients who have had a heart attack and been given statin therapy have a second attack, while others do not? The answer is that people *vary*. People have different body characteristics (e.g., weight, blood pressure and blood measurements), genetic make-up and lifestyles (e.g., diet, exercise, and smoking and alcohol consumption habits). These lead to **variability** or **natural variation.** People respond to the same exposure or treatment in different ways. When a new intervention is evaluated, it is essential to consider whether the observed responses are consistent with natural variation (i.e. chance) or whether there really is a treatment effect. This is a principal concern of medical statistics.

1.4 Alternatives to clinical trials

Examining interventions can be done using a clinical trial and in particular a randomised controlled trial (RCT), observational study or trial with historical controls. They have fundamentally different designs. Some observational studies are used as supporting evidence for the effectiveness and safety of an intervention under the topic **real-world evidence** (RWE) or **real-world data** (RWD); see Chapter 9.

Although studies other than RCTs can provide useful information about an intervention, care is needed over their interpretation. Observational studies, for example, can give the same or conflicting conclusion to RCTs:

- A review of 20 observational studies indicated that giving the influenza vaccine to the elderly could halve the risk of developing respiratory and flu-like symptoms.[4] Practically the same effect was found in a large double-blind RCT.[5]
- A review of 6 observational studies indicated that people with a high β-carotene intake, by eating lots of fruit and vegetables, had a 31% reduction in the risk of cardiovascular death than those with a low intake.[6] However, 4 RCTs together showed that a high intake increases the risk by 12%.[6]

Observational (non-randomised) studies

Observational studies may be useful in evaluating treatments with large effects, although there may still be uncertainty over the actual size of the effec.[7, 8] They can have a larger number of participants than RCTs and therefore provide more evidence on side effects,

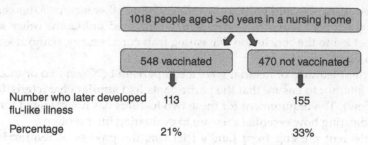

Figure 1.2 Example of an observational study of the flu vaccine. Source: Adapted from[9].

particularly uncommon ones. However, when the treatment effect is small or moderate, the potential design limitations of observational studies can make it difficult to establish whether a new intervention is truly effective. These limitations are called **confounding** and **bias**.

Several observational studies have examined the effect of the influenza vaccine in preventing flu and respiratory disease in elderly individuals. Such a study would involve taking a group of people aged over 60 years, then ascertaining whether each participant had had the influenza vaccine or not, and who subsequently developed flu or flu-like illnesses. An example is given in Figure 1.2.[9] The chance of developing flu-like illness was lower in the vaccine group than in the unvaccinated group: 21 versus 33%. However, did the flu vaccine really work?

Assume that vitamin C protects against acquiring influenza. People who choose to have the vaccine might also happen to eat more fruit than those who are unvaccinated (Table 1.1). The difference in flu rates of 5 versus 10% could be due to the vaccine only, the difference in fruit intake (80 vs 15%) only or both together. But we are not interested in fruit intake. If fruit intake had not been measured, it could be incorrectly concluded that the difference in flu rates is due to the vaccination.

When the association between an intervention (e.g. flu vaccine) and a disorder (e.g. flu) is examined, a spurious relationship could be created through a third factor, called a **confounding factor** (e.g. eating fruit). A confounder needs to be correlated with both the intervention *and* the disorder of interest. Even though there are methods of design and analysis that can allow for their effects, there could exist unknown confounders for which no adjustment can be made because they were not measured. There is also **residual confounding** which occurs when the statistical adjustment for a confounder has been insufficient.

There may also be **bias**, where the actions of participants or researchers produce a value of the trial endpoint that is *systematically* under- or over-reported in one trial group. In the flu example, the clinician or carer could deliberately choose fitter people to be vaccinated,

Table 1.1 Hypothetical observational study of the flu vaccine.

	1000 people aged ≥60 years	
	Vaccinated N = 200	*Not vaccinated N = 800*
Eat fruit regularly	160 (80%)	120 (15%)
Developed flu	10 (5%)	80 (10%)

Box 1.1 Confounding and bias

Confounding represents the natural relationships between the physical and biochemical characteristics, genetic make-up and lifestyle/behavioural habits that may affect how an individual responds to a treatment.

- It cannot be removed from a research study, but known confounders can be measured and therefore allowed for in a statistical analysis.

Bias is a study design feature that affects how participants are selected, treated, managed or assessed, which systematically distorts the results in one trial group more than another.

- It can be prevented, but human nature sometimes makes this difficult.
- It is difficult to allow for bias in statistical analyses because it often cannot be measured.

Randomisation within a clinical trial minimises the effect of confounding and some biases.

---

believing they would benefit the most. Also, the vaccinated group may be people who chose to go to their family doctor and request the vaccine. It is therefore possible that people who were vaccinated had different lifestyles and characteristics than unvaccinated people. The effect of the vaccine could be over-estimated if the vaccinated people are less likely to acquire the flu than the unvaccinated ones.

When designing trials, it is a useful exercise to imagine being a participant, someone who allocates/administers the trial interventions, or someone who assesses outcome measures, and consider whether there is anything that can be done that can distort the results. Then consider how this could be minimised or avoided by the trial design and conduct.

Confounding is sometimes called a form of bias because both affect the results. However, it is useful to distinguish them (Box 1.1).

1.5 Types of clinical trials

Clinical trials are broadly categorised into four types (Phase I, II, III and IV), largely depending on the main aim (Box 1.2).

Phase I	Phase II	Phase III	Phase IV (real-world data)
Safety/toxicity	*Efficacy*	*Efficacy*	Effectiveness
Pharmacology	Safety	Safety	Long term safety
	Adherence	Adherence	Uncommon side effects
		Quality of life	New indications
		Health economics	

Words in italics indicate the common primary focus.

Efficacy and effectiveness are used interchangeably. However, efficacy is sometimes used in a clinical trial setting where the participants could be a select (often motivated) group with high adherence to the trial intervention. Effectiveness applies to routine practice, which better reflects the use of the treatment in the target group and the extent of adherence among them. The magnitude of benefit associated with a new therapy is sometimes higher when using efficacy than effectiveness.

Traditionally, there has been a sequence from phase I to phase III involving separate trials, particularly for pharmaceutical drugs. To reduce the entire evaluation period, phases can be combined within the same protocol (for example, phase I/II or phase II/III).

Box 1.2 Types of trials

Phase I

- First time a new drug or regimen is examined in humans ('first-in-human' studies), and also used to examine a licenced drug for a new indication (disorder) or a new combination of therapies.
- Few participants (often <50 but can sometimes be >100 if covering multiple disease subtypes).
- Primary aims: check that the toxicity profile is acceptable; find a dose (e.g. drug or radiotherapy) that is tolerable; examine the biological and pharmacological effects.
- Patients or healthy volunteers are monitored closely.

Phase II

Often 30–100 people (but may be larger in common disorders).
- Aims to obtain a *preliminary* estimate of efficacy and further evidence of harms.
- May be single group or randomised (multiple groups), including a control therapy.
- Results are used to help design a confirmatory phase III trial; or the efficacy evidence is good enough to change practice for rare disorders or when there is clear unmet need

Phase III

- Should (must) be randomised and with a comparison (control) group.
- Relatively large (usually several hundred or thousand people).
- Aims to provide a *definitive* answer on whether a new treatment is better than the control group (**superiority**), or similarly effective (**equivalence**) or not materially worse (**non-inferiority**) but with other advantages
- Used to obtain a marketing authorisation from a regulatory agency or for market access for a new drug or medical device (pivotal trial).

Phase IV (post-marketing, surveillance or real-world studies).

- Relatively large (usually several hundred or thousand people).
- Used to continue to monitor efficacy and safety in the population once the new treatment has been adopted into routine practice.
- Not usually randomised, but there are pragmatic randomised phase IV studies that compare currently used interventions.
- Based on participants in the general target population, rather than the selected group who agreed to participate in a phase III trial.

1.6 Key design features

Clinical trials have common fundamental design characteristics (Figure 1.3).

Inclusion and exclusion criteria

Specifying which participants are recruited is done using an **eligibility list**: a set of **inclusion and exclusion** criteria which each participant has to fulfil before they can take part. Common criteria include age range, having no serious co-morbid conditions, the ability to give consent, having no known contraindications to the therapy, and no previous or recent exposure to the trial treatment or others that are similar to it. They should have unambiguous definitions to make recruiting participants easier.

Having many criteria produces a homogenous group that is more likely to respond to the treatment in a similar manner, making it easier to detect an effect if it exists, particularly small or moderate effects. However, the trial results might not be easily generalisable. A trial with few criteria will have greater generalisability but more variability, perhaps making it more difficult to show that the treatment is effective and sometimes only large effects can be detected easily.

Studies increasingly use biomarkers or molecular/genetic testing (profiling) of blood, urine or tissue samples to select only patients who are more likely to benefit from a new treatment that has been developed specifically for that type of patient (**precision/personalised medicine**).

Experimental/investigational treatment group

The new intervention could have been developed using prior studies or laboratory research. Importantly, its description and delivery should be clear enough for other people to replicate it. Investigators expect to show that a new intervention is more effective than the control group (**superiority**), or it has an effect that is similar (**equivalence**) or 'not much worse' (**non-inferiority**).

Control (comparator) group

The outcome of participants given the new intervention can be compared with that in a control group. A **control** group normally receives the current standard of care, no intervention or placebo (see Blinding below). Treatment effects from RCTs are therefore always comparative. The choice of the control intervention depends on the availability of alternative treatments, what is recommended in local or national clinical guidelines, or the requirements of regulatory agencies or organisations responsible for market access. When an established treatment exists, it can be unethical to give a placebo instead because this deprives some participants of a known benefit.

Randomisation and allocating participants

The randomisation process ensures that each participant has the same chance of being allocated to a group as everyone else (Box 1.3). Neither the participant or research team can influence which intervention is given. This minimises the effect of both known *and unknown* confounders, and thus has a distinct advantage over observational studies in which statistical adjustments can only be made for known confounders that have been measured. Randomisation does not produce *identical* groups; there will always be small differences because of chance variation.

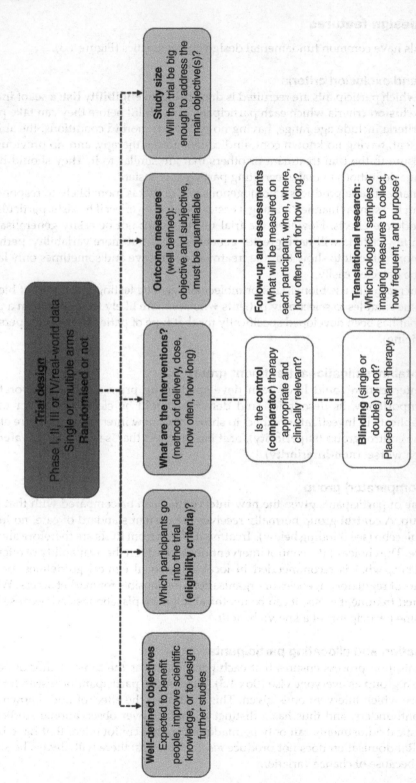

Figure 1.3 Overview of trial design features. Examples of objectives are: "To determine whether Intervention A reduces the risk of dying among people who have had a stroke"; "To evaluate whether Therapy B is non-inferior to standard of care in people with chronic lung disease"; "To investigate whether Drug A has potential efficacy and acceptable toxicities in patients with multiple sclerosis".

Box 1.3 'Make everything the same' except the interventions: randomisation

• If the trial groups being compared have fundamental different characteristics, behaviours and disease features (confounding and bias), it is not easy to determine whether an experimental intervention has been effective or not.
• The most reliable approach to evaluate an intervention is to make the trial groups *the same*.
• Randomly allocating participants produces groups that are similar with regard to all characteristics *except the trial interventions*.
• The only systematic difference between the two groups should be the treatment given.
• Therefore, the trial results should only be due to the effect of the new treatment i.e. confounding or bias have not spuriously produced or hidden an effect.
• In addition to ensuring baseline characteristics are similar, how participants are managed, followed up and assessed should also be the same between the trial arms to avoid/minimise bias.

Randomisation minimises confounding and some bias. Examples of bias are:
• **Selection bias** can occur if choosing a particular participant for the trial is influenced by knowing the next treatment allocation.
• **Allocation bias** involves giving the trial treatment that the investigator or participant feels might be most beneficial. This can be avoided if randomisation is done through a central office or computer system because the researcher has no control over the process (called **allocation concealment**).
Random number lists can be generated using, for example Microsoft Excel; there are commercial or freely available software that perform randomisations; or someone with computing skills can create a bespoke system. Box 1.4 shows randomisation methods. Many investigators use 1:1 allocation (half the individuals receive the experimental intervention, and half receive the control intervention). In some cases, unequal allocation (e.g. 2:1) is used, in order to get more information, such as side effects, about the new intervention.

The choice of method depends on the size of the trial and number of stratification factors. Simple randomisation or permuted block randomisation should produce well-balanced characteristics in very large trials (several thousand). Stratified randomisation using permuted blocks is acceptable if the investigators wish to use random numbers and there are few (prognostic) stratification factors. But in small trials (e.g. <100 participants) or when many factors are used, this method could produce groups where one or more factors are noticeably imbalanced by chance. Minimisation handles several stratification factors easily.

Outcome measures (endpoints) and collecting data
An **outcome measure** (**endpoint**) is something that enables a disorder, symptom or risk factor to be quantified. Outcome measures can reflect efficacy (benefits), harms, health-related quality of life and adherence.

Phase I trials will have several outcome measures usually with a focus on adverse events. Most phase II and III trials typically have one to three **primary endpoints**[#]

[#] Generally used to justify a change in practice or further studies.

Box 1.4 Methods for allocating participants within RCTs

Random allocation

• **Simple randomisation**: analogous to tossing a coin (heads: Treatment A; tails: Treatment B). In reality a randomly generated list of numbers between 0 and 9 is used: give Treatment A if 0 to 4, and Treatment B if 5 to 9.

• **Permuted block randomisation**: simple randomisation performed using varying even-numbered block sizes to achieve complete balance in each block (e.g. with block size 6, there will be three participants given Treatment A and three given Treatment B).

• **Stratified randomisation**: either of the above methods are used within each level of at least one (stratification) factor known to be strongly associated with the trial outcomes. Investigators want to be assured that these factors are well balanced (e.g. with sex, there are separate randomisation lists for men and women, ensuring a similar number of men and women appear in each trial group).

Dynamic allocation or minimisation

• **Minimisation** also ensures balance for several factors. The treatment allocation for the first few participants (e.g. 20) can be made using simple randomisation. Then the allocation for each subsequent participant depends on the distribution of the stratification factors among those who have already been randomised: e.g. if there are more patients already allocated to Treatment A, the method allocates the next person to Treatment B.

• Minimisation is sometimes considered to not reflect true randomisation because it does not use random numbers. This is addressed by using a high probability (80 or 90%) of being allocated to the next treatment, instead of with certainty.

• Minimisation should not be used for single centre trials.

What matters is that it is not possible for anyone to predict or influence the next treatment allocation: randomness = unpredictability.

(considered the most important and clinically relevant), each corresponding to a **primary objective**. There are also several **secondary endpoints** and **objectives** (considered as supporting evidence), and perhaps some exploratory endpoints. There are five key areas of outcome measures (see Box 2.1, page 16).

Outcome measures come from various sources (Box 1.5). In many situations, there will already be established key endpoints (e.g., the occurrence of coronary heart disease and stroke in type 2 diabetes). In other areas such as in Alzheimer's disease and dementia, there may be no single established primary endpoint because there is an array of imaging tests and clinical assessments. For chronic disorders such as depression, respiratory lung disease and psoriasis, the outcomes need to reflect patient-relevant changes in symptoms due to the new intervention.

Collecting data electronically is increasingly used. Participants enter their own data in real time using personal electronic devices at home, instead of staying longer in clinics to complete paper forms. Many hospitals use electronic records so patient and outcome data can be extracted from those systems; and several countries have regional or national databases and registries that contain outcomes such as cancer occurrence and deaths.

Box 1.5 Sources of data

- Case report forms completed by research staff
- Face-to-face or telephone interviews with participants
- Self-completed questionnaires (handed or posted back to the researchers)
- Face-to-face interviews or questionnaires completed by a proxy for the study participant (e.g. carer or relative)
- Personal electronic devices (mobile phones, apps, internet weblinks and wearables)
- Biological samples (e.g. blood, urine, saliva or tissue)
- Imaging tests (e.g. X-ray, ultrasound, CT, PET or MRI scans)
- Health records from family or primary care clinics, or hospitals
- Local, regional or national registries/databases* that routinely record population data on, for example deaths and cause of death, occurrence of a disorder or how a specific disorder is treated and managed. Trial participants would need to be 'linked' to these databases.

*These can come from governmental, commercial or academic institutions.

Blinding (placebo)

Randomisation minimises some bias, but not all. Participants and researchers often have expectations associated with a particular treatment that affect how people respond to it, or how the researcher manages or assesses them. In participants, this bias is called the **placebo effect**: the psychological ability to affect their own health status. The effect of bias could result in participants who receive the new intervention appearing to do better than the control group, but the difference is not really due to the action of the new treatment.

Clinical trials are described as **double-blind** if neither the participant nor anyone involved in giving the treatment, or managing or assessing the participant, is aware of which treatment was given. In **single-blind** trials, usually only the participant is blind to the treatment he/she has received, but occasionally the participant is aware but the assessor is blind to treatment.

A placebo has no known active component. It could be a tablet, capsule, saline injection, sham surgical procedure, sham medical device or any other intervention that is meant to resemble the experimental intervention, but it has no known effect on the disorder of interest.

An example illustrating the importance of placebos comes from a trial of patients with osteoarthritis of the knee. At the time, such patients often underwent knee surgery (arthroscopic lavage or débridement). Patients typically reported less pain afterwards but there was no clear biological rationale for this. A single-blinded randomised trial[10] comparing these two surgical procedures with sham surgery (skin incision to the knee) provided no evidence that they reduced knee pain.

Using placebos needs to be justified in any clinical trial, approved by an independent ethics board, and participants are fully aware that they may be assigned to the sham group.

When blinding is not possible, it is best to use outcome measures that do not rely on human judgement. For example, in a trial evaluating hypnotherapy for smoking cessation, a **subjective endpoint** would be to ask participants whether they stopped smoking at 1 year. However, some continuing smokers deliberately misreport their smoking status, leading to bias. An **objective endpoint** would be to measure urinary cotinine, as a marker of current smoking status, which is specific to tobacco smoke inhalation and less prone to bias than self-reported habits.

Participant follow-up

Once participants enrol in a trial, outcome measures must be obtained directly from them and/or via health records. The type and timing of assessments which produce the endpoints should be:
- similar between the trial groups (to avoid bias) when possible;
- able to detect changes in the disorder at clinically important time points that reflect its natural history (e.g., assessments could be frequent early on for trials of advanced/acute disorders, or infrequent for preventive trials when the disorder can take years to occur); and
- pragmatic, where possible, to reflect routine practice, and not be arduous for participants or local research staff by requiring too many extra clinic visits or tests.

Following are examples of bias that may occur:

Withdrawal bias: participants in one trial group are more likely to withdraw from the study than other arms (e.g. due to side effects).

Follow-up bias: there is less follow-up on one trial arm than another, or the reasons for lack of follow-up are very different between the arms and associated with the trial interventions.

Study size

Justifying how large a trial needs to be is an important component of a grant application or review by an ethics board or regulatory agency. Phase I and II trials tend to be relatively small, while phase III trials must be large enough to provide a clear answer. It is better to have an overly large study than one that is not quite big enough which produces equivocal results from which no clear recommendation can be made (resources could then have been wasted).

There is nothing wrong with small trials as long as they are well-designed and conducted. They can be quick and relatively cheap, only require a few centres and produce an answer in a short time frame. This avoids spending too many resources on looking for a treatment effect when there really is none. However, if a positive result is found a larger confirmatory study is often needed.

Contrary to common belief, sample size estimation is not an exact science. If the target is 100 patients, researchers often believe that recruiting 95 or 105 is a problem: it is not. Sample sizes provide an *approximate* trial size to aim for, and reaching a few less or more than the target is not an issue at all.

Translational research (bio- and imaging markers)

There have been major technological advances in laboratory and imaging techniques, including cheaper and quicker genetic sequencing of normal and abnormal cells (e.g. cancer). This has led to the discovery of many biomarkers measured in tissue, blood, serum, skin, urine and saliva, and markers from imaging methods using modern and sophisticated CT, PET and MRI scans. The marker could be a biochemical measure in biospecimens, familial genetic trait or abnormality (germline), or genetic abnormality/mutation in for example tumour tissue or circulating tumour cells (somatic). New treatments have thus been developed and evaluated in clinical trials that are targeted to a specific marker measured at baseline (i.e. before treatment), in which patients with the marker (e.g. their cancer cells have a particular genetic mutation) benefit much more than with standard (non-targeted therapies). This is the fundamental premise of **precision (personalised or risk-stratified) medicine**, i.e. there is no longer a 'one-size-fits-all' approach to treating several disorders but instead subsets of patients derive greater benefit from treatments that target a specific feature (marker) of their disease. Biomarker-driven trials will become more common as we obtain a greater biological understanding of various disorders, including how they develop and their natural history. They can be used for:

- correlative science
- biomarker discovery
- prognostic and predictive markers
- genomics
- identifying drug resistance
- disease monitoring

Biomarkers can be used to determine eligibility for a trial and also which trial treatment a person receives, or they can be evaluated at the end of the study to see if outcomes are influenced by the marker (**predictive marker**). Biomarkers can also be used to gain a better understanding of the mechanisms of action of a new therapy or evaluated to see whether they can be used to forecast patient prognosis or outcomes (**prognostic marker**).

Several funding organisations expect planned translational research to be included within a clinical trial proposal.

1.7 Summary points

- Clinical trials are essential for evaluating new methods of disease detection, prevention and treatment.
- Observational studies can provide useful supporting evidence on the effectiveness and safety of an intervention, but they have limitations.
- Clinical trials, especially when randomised, are considered to provide the strongest evidence.
- Randomisation minimises the effect of confounding and bias, and blinding further reduces the potential for bias.
- Understand the key design features: Participants/Population, Intervention, Control and Outcome measures (PICO).
- PPIE should be used to help design, conduct and interpret trials.
- Translational research (measurement of bio- and imaging markers) can play an important role in precision medicine as well as understanding mechanisms of action and predicting patient outcomes.

References

1. Hackshaw AK. *A concise guide to observational studies*. 1st edn, Wiley-Blackwell, 2015.
2. https://www.jameslindlibrary.org/lind-j-1753/
3. Medical Research Council. Streptomycin treatment of pulmonary tuberculosis. *BMJ* 1948; 2:769–782.

4. Gross PA, Hermogenes H, Sacks HS, Lau J, Levandowski RA. The efficacy of influenza vaccine in elderly persons. *Ann Intern Med* 1995; **123**:518–527.

5. Govaert TME, Thijs CTMCN, Masurel N *et al*. The efficacy of influenza vaccination in elderly individuals. *JAMA* 1994; **272**(21):1661–1665.

6. Egger M, Schneider M, Davey Smith G. Meta-analysis: spurious precision? Meta-analysis of observational studies. *BMJ* 1998; **316**:140–144.

7. Collins R, MacMahon S. Reliable assessment of the effects of treatment on mortality and major morbidity, I: clinical trials. *Lancet* 2001; **357**:373–380.

8. MacMahon S, Collins R. Reliable assessment of the effects of treatment on mortality and major morbidity, II: observational studies. *Lancet* 2001; **357**:455–462.

9. Patriarca PA, Weber JA, Parker RA *et al*. Efficacy of influenza vaccine in nursing homes. Reduction in illness and complications during an influenza A (H3N2) epidemic. *JAMA* 1985; **253**:1136–1139.

10. Moseley JB, O'Malley K, Petersen NJ *et al*. A controlled trial of arthroscopic surgery for osteoarthritis of the knee. *N Engl J Med* 2002; **347**(2):81–88.

CHAPTER 2

Types of outcome measures and understanding them

It is essential that we can *quantify* the benefits and harms of a new therapy so that healthy people, patients and health professionals can make informed decisions about a new intervention. This chapter provides an overview of the basic principles of outcome measures.

2.1 Clinical trial outcome measures (endpoints)

Features of 'good' outcome measures include:
- Clearly defined and quantifiable
- Easily/readily measurable and reproducible
- Unaffected by bias
- Clinically relevant to patients/individuals
- Reflects impacts on well-being and personal costs
- Reflects impacts on society (e.g. ability to work)
- Clinically relevant to health professionals.

They could also provide major new insights into how a new treatment works (e.g. bio- or imaging markers). Many outcome measures are already established by the medical community, or accepted by regulatory and reimbursement/health technology assessment agencies for practice changing trials of drugs and medical devices.

There are several areas of outcome measures (Box 2.1). The specific choice of efficacy endpoints depends on the trial objectives (e.g. prevent a disorder, improve/maintain symptoms, prolong survival).

Although these measures tend to be reported separately, they can be correlated. Severe side effects could lead to stopping the trial treatment early (low adherence), and then ultimately lower efficacy because of insufficient exposure to get the full benefits.

Harms (adverse events) are essential to record and report. Few interventions have no adverse events at all. When interpreting adverse events, consider:
- Whether they are symptomatic or asymptomatic (the latter includes abnormal biochemical measures)
- Severity (which may affect adults and children differently; and people with acute versus chronic disorders tolerate adverse events and their severity differently)
- Whether the events are easily treated, prevented or managed; and the cost of this
- Whether the events occur repeatedly in a person
- Whether the events interfere with the person's daily living and ability to work and function.

A Concise Guide to Clinical Trials, Second Edition. Allan Hackshaw.
© 2024 John Wiley & Sons Ltd. Published 2024 by John Wiley & Sons Ltd.

Box 2.1 Five areas of clinical trial outcome measures

1. Efficacy — Measures (clinical) benefit

2. Safety (side effects, adverse events, toxicity) — Measures harm

3. Adherence (compliance) to the experimental or control interventions, or background standard therapies given at the same time — Do people continue to take the interventions as planned or do they stop early? If they stop early, why?

4. Patient/participant reported outcomes — Measure health-related quality of life, well-being and other things that matter to patients

5. Biomarkers (translational research)* — Obtain new biological insights about the mechanism of action of a new treatment; find a prognostic marker (that can forecast outcomes for a participant) or a predictive marker (that can identify which participants would or would not benefit from a therapy)

*Measured not only during and after treatment but also at baseline (pre-treatment), where it would not strictly be an outcome measure but rather a baseline characteristic.

Health-related quality of life (QoL) measures can reflect benefit (efficacy) or harm, but as they are subjective (self-reported measures) they are often considered separately from clinical endpoints. For some chronic disorders, QoL is the primary endpoint.

Adherence is often focused on the trial interventions, but adherence to other (standard) treatments given at the same time as the trial therapies is similarly important but sometimes overlooked. If the experimental therapy has side effects that lead to patients suspending or stopping (effective) standard treatment early, this can negatively impact patients.

2.2 'True' versus surrogate outcome measures

Many outcome measures have an obvious and direct clinical impact on participants, for example, whether they:
- Die (i.e. die earlier than expected)
- Develop a symptomatic disease/disorder
- Reflect important components of quality of life.

These are sometimes referred to as **true or hard endpoints**, because the person can see or feel it, or an observer can see the impact of it (e.g. death). A clear benefit of statins is

---

Box 2.2 Examples of true and surrogate trial endpoints

Surrogate endpoint	True endpoint
Low-density lipoprotein (LDL) cholesterol level	Heart attack and stroke
Blood pressure	Stroke
Tumour size or time to cancer progression	Overall survival
CD4 count or RNA viral load	Death from AIDS
Intra-ocular pressure	Glaucoma

---

evident in a clinical trial where the outcome measure is a cardiovascular event such as stroke or heart attack. For several disorders, there is the concept of a **surrogate endpoint (marker)**.[1-4] A surrogate marker ideally should be a good predictor of a 'hard' endpoint, where they are closely correlated via some biological process; or it identifies a person at increased risk of the hard endpoint.

Surrogate outcomes tend to be measurements from biospecimens or imaging tests (Box 2.2) so they are sometimes not considered to be 'clinically relevant'. For example, if a tumour grows by 2 mm or a brain scan shows a plaque lesion has increased by 3 mm (Alzheimer's disease), the person usually cannot feel it or their health management does not change.

Sometimes, a trial using a hard endpoint would have to be large or take many years to conduct. Therefore the appeal of surrogate outcomes is that they:
- are measured sooner than a hard endpoint
- are often more sensitive in response to a treatment
- have more events, requiring smaller, shorter, or cheaper trials.

Treatment trials for people newly diagnosed with HIV usually just need to show that RNA viral load can be kept very low or undetectable as a measure of efficacy. In other diseases, it is often difficult to find good surrogates, and there is controversy over their use. While surrogate measures may be used in early phase trials as initial signs of treatment activity, they are sometimes not accepted as primary endpoints in definitive phase III trials unless they have been validated, or there is an accepted biological or clinical link between the surrogate and hard endpoints.

Technological advances in biomarkers and imaging means that more surrogate markers are likely to become available for several disorders. However, they need careful consideration if proposed as primary outcome measures. For example, in two trials of aducanumab for treating early-stage Alzheimer's disease, the large reduction in amyloid plaque measured by PET scans did not lead to large benefits on cognition and function (Box 2.3).[5]

When evaluating a new drug or medical device, regulatory authorities and health technology assessment agencies sometimes have guidance on acceptable surrogate markers.[4]

Box 2.3 Effect of high dose aducanumab on the change in surrogate or hard endpoints from baseline to week 78. Source: Budd Haeberlein et al.[5]

	Surrogate endpoint Amyloid plaque (PET scan)	Hard endpoint Composite of cognition and function*
EMERGE trial	71% decrease ($p < 0.001$)	0.03 increase ($p = 0.83$) No evidence of benefit
ENGAGE trial	59% decrease ($p < 0.001$)	0.39 decrease ($p = 0.01$) Statistically significant but a small clinical effect

*Using the Clinical Dementia Rating-Sum of Boxes (CDR-SB) score (range 0–18). A decrease in score from baseline represents benefit.

2.3 Types of outcomes

All outcome measures fall into three basic categories:
- **counting people (categorical data)**
- **taking measurements on people (continuous data)**
- **time-to-event data**.

Distinguishing between them helps to define the trial objectives, methods of sample size calculation and statistical analysis, and interpreting and communicating the results.

First, the **unit of interest** is determined, usually a person. Second, consider what will be done to the unit of interest. The outcome measure will involve either **counting** how many people have a particular characteristic (i.e. put them into mutually exclusive groups, such as 'dead' or 'alive') or **taking measurements** on them. In some situations, taking a measurement on someone involves counting something, but the unit of interest is still a person. For **time-to-event** data, we have to define the event (e.g. death); then we measure the *time* it takes for each person to reach the event (e.g. time until death). Examples of these outcome measures are shown in Figure 6.1, page 80).

When measuring an endpoint for each trial participant, we have many data values and it is impossible for us to interpret them at once. Therefore, we turn all of these values into one or two numbers using **summary statistics** that allow us to better understand the data and communicate the findings to others. Further details can be found in books on medical statistics.[6,7] Sections 2.4 to 2.6 show how data are summarized for one group of people. Other summary statistics are used for comparing two groups (called **effect sizes**), and these are covered in Chapter 6.

When using summary statistics, we refer to an *average* treatment effect in a group of participants and do not usually predict response to treatment for an individual.

2.4 Counting people

This type of outcome measure is easily summarised by calculating the **percentage** or **proportion** in each category. For example, the effect of a flu vaccine can be examined by counting how many people developed flu in the vaccinated group in a trial, and dividing this number by the total number of patients in that group. This proportion (or percentage) is the **risk**, i.e. the risk of developing flu if vaccinated. The same calculation is made in the unvaccinated group, i.e. the risk of developing flu if not vaccinated. In Figure 1.2 (page 4) (the two risks are 21 and 33%. The word 'risk' implies something negative, but it could be used for any outcome that involves counting people, for example, the risk of being alive after 5 years, or the risk of being discharged from hospital by 30 days. However, these sound strange so we can use the word 'chance' instead of 'risk'.

2.5 Taking measurements on people

This type of outcome measure varies between people. It is often used for chronic disorders (e.g. to show changes in disease symptoms over time), health-related quality of life and biomarkers.

Consider the following cholesterol levels (mmol/L) for 40 healthy men, all aged 45 years (ranked in order of size):

3.6	3.8	3.9	4.1	4.2	4.5	4.5	4.8	5.1	5.3
5.4	5.4	5.6	5.8	5.9	6.0	6.1	6.1	6.2	6.3
6.4	6.5	6.6	6.8	6.9	7.1	7.2	7.2	7.3	7.4
7.5	7.7	8.0	8.1	8.1	8.2	8.3	9.0	9.1	10.0

These data are summarised by two parameters: the 'average' level and a measure of spread or variability. The average, often referred to as a measure of central tendency, is usually described by either the **mean** or the **median**. It is where the middle of the distribution lies. Some people interpret this as a 'typical' value when trying to use layman's terms to describe central tendency. The mean is more commonly reported and often taken to be the same as the average.

The mean is the sum of all the values divided by the number of observations. In the example above, the mean is $256/40 = 6.4$ mmol/L. The median is the value that has half the observations above it and half below. In the example, it is halfway between the 20th and 21st values; median $= (6.3+6.4)/2 = 6.35$ mmol/L.

One measure of spread is the **standard deviation**. It quantifies variability, i.e. how much the data spreads about from the mean. It is calculated as:

$$\sqrt{\frac{\text{Sum of (the distances of each data point from the mean)}^2}{(\text{Number of data values} - 1)}}$$

In the example of 40 men, the standard deviation is 1.57 mmol/L: the cholesterol levels differ from the mean value of 6.4 by, on average, 1.57 mmol/L.

Another measure of spread is **the interquartile range**. This is the difference between the 25th centile (the value that has a quarter of the data below it and three-quarters above it) and the 75th centile (the value that has three-quarters of the data below it and a quarter above it). In the example, there are 40 observations so the 25th centile is between the 10th and 11th data points (i.e. 5.32 mmol/L) and the 75th centile is between the 30th and 31st data

Cholesterol (mmol/L)	Number of men	Percentage
3.0–3.9	3	7.5
4.0–4.9	5	12.5
5.0–5.9	7	17.5
6.0–6.9	10	25.0
7.0–7.9	7	17.5
8.0–8.9	5	12.5
9.0–9.9	2	5.0
10.0–10.9	1	2.5
Total	40	100.0

Table 2.1 Frequency distribution of cholesterol levels of a sample of 40 men (page 21).

points (i.e. 7.47 mmol/L).[#] The interquartile range is therefore 7.47 − 5.32 = 2.15 mmol/L. Sometimes, the actual 25th and 75th centiles are presented instead of the interquartile range.

Deciding which measures of average and spread to use depends on whether the distribution is symmetric or not. To help determine this, the data are grouped into categories of cholesterol levels and the **frequency distribution** is examined (Table 2.1). These proportions are used to create a **histogram** (the shaded boxes in Figure 2.1). The shape is reasonably symmetric, indicating that the distribution is **Gaussian** or **Normal** ('N' is in capital letters to avoid confusion with the usual definition of the word normal, which can indicate people without disease). This is more easily visualised by drawing a curve around the histogram (Figure 2.1), which is said to be bell-shaped.

When data are Normally distributed, the mean and median are similar. The preferred measures of average and spread are the mean and standard deviation, because they have useful mathematical properties, which underlie many statistical methods of analysis. When the data are not Normally distributed, other measures are used. Consider the outcome measure 'number of days in hospital' for 20 patients, where the histogram is shown in Figure 2.2, and it is clearly not symmetric. The data are **skewed to the right** (there is a long tail at the right). When most of the data are towards the right, the distribution is said

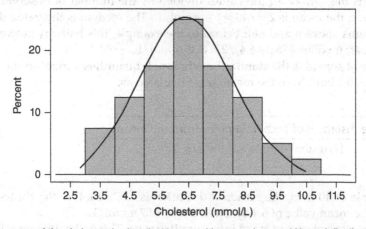

Figure 2.1 Histogram of the cholesterol values in 40 men, with a superimposed Normal distribution curve.

[#] The 25th centile is the point at $(n + 1)/4$, i.e. the 10.25th observation. This is between the 10th and 11th value, i.e. 5.3 and 5.4, and found by adding 0.25 × difference between these two observations (0.1) to 5.3. So the 25th centile is 5.3 + 0.025 = 5.325. A similar calculation is made to obtain the 75th centile.

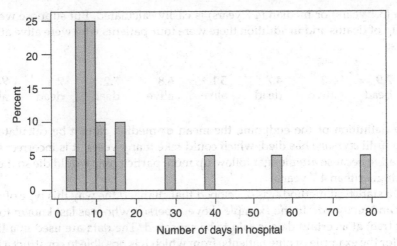

Figure 2.2 Histogram of the length of hospital stay for 20 patients.

to be **skewed to the left**. The middle of the data and spread are better represented by the median and interquartile range. The mean and standard deviation are heavily influenced by the few very high values.

The summary statistics that describe these data are:

Mean = 17 days   Standard deviation = 19 days
Median = 9 days   Interquartile range = 8 days

When data are skewed, it is sometimes possible to **transform** them, usually by taking **logarithms** or the **square root**. Many biological measurements only have a Normal (symmetric) distribution on a logarithmic scale, so using the log of the values produces a symmetric histogram as in Figure 2.1. The mean is calculated using the log of the values, and the result is back-transformed to the original scale, though this cannot be done with standard deviation. For example, if the mean of the transformed values is 0.81, using log to the base 10, the calculation $10^{0.81} = 6.5$ produces the mean value on the original scale. This is called a **geometric mean**. Sometimes no transformation is possible that will turn a skewed distribution into a Normal one. In these situations, the median and interquartile range could be used. A probability (or centile) plot can be used to determine whether data are Normally distributed or not. Many statistical software packages provide this.

Regardless of which measures of average and spread are used, it is important to realise that summarising data is imperfect. In the cholesterol example, the mean of 6.4 mmol/L cannot tell us about the whole range of values. Although the typical value for the 40 men is 6.4, some have levels that are exactly 6.4 while others have levels above or below this.

2.6 Time-to-event measures

Here, an event could be defined in many ways, and one of the most commonly used is 'death', hence the term **survival analysis**. Other definitions of an event are given in Box 2.4. In the following five patients, the endpoint is defined as 'time from randomisation until death (in years)', and all have died:

2.7   2.9   4.7   7.2   7.8

The mean (5.1 years) or median (4.7 years) is easily calculated. But suppose we had the same group of deaths and in addition there were four patients who were alive at the time of analysis:

2.7	2.9	3.3	4.7	5.1	6.8	7.2	7.8	9.1
dead	dead	alive	dead	alive	alive	dead	dead	alive

Given the definition of the endpoint, the mean or median cannot be calculated in the usual way until *everyone* has died, which could take many years. It is incorrect to ignore those still alive because after longer follow-up more participants would die so the median would be higher than 4.7 years.

In 1958, a statistical method was developed that changed the way this type of data was displayed and analysed.[8] In the example above, a person who was last known to be alive (i.e. event free) at a certain date is said to be **censored**. The data are used in a **life-table** (Table 2.2 for the example of nine patients) from which it is possible to construct a **Kaplan–Meier plot** (Figure 2.3). This approach uses the last available information on every person and how long he/she has lived for, or has been in the study.

Every time a participant has an event (here, dies), the step drops down (the first drop is at 2.7 years). When participants are censored, four in the example, they contribute no further information to the analysis after the censoring date. The plot appears as a smooth curve when there are many events.

Censoring is as important as events.[#] There are several reasons why participants could be censored: they truly have not had the event yet, they are lost to follow-up (e.g. moved away/abroad), they have not had their last assessment yet, or they have had a recent assessment but this information has not yet been passed to the trial investigators. Reasons for censoring should be unrelated to the study and trial

Table 2.2 Survival data of the example of nine patients. The last column is plotted against the first column to produce a Kaplan–Meier curve.

Time since randomisation (years)	1 = dead, i.e. event 0= censored (no event yet)	Number of patients at risk	Percentage alive (survival rate %)
0	–	9	100
2.7	1	9	89
2.9	1	8	78
3.3	0	7	78
4.7	1	6	65
5.1	0	5	65
6.8	0	4	65
7.2	1	3	43
7.8	1	2	22
9.1	0	1	22

- The last column comes from a formula which uses the number at risk at each time point and the risk of dying in the previous time interval.
- 5-year survival rate is the value at exactly 5 years or the closest value just below 5 (i.e. 65%).
- Median survival is the point at which 50% of patients are alive or the closest value just below which is 43% (median is 7.2 years).

[#] Dates when participants are censored should always be clearly defined and acceptable (e.g., date last seen, date of stopping treatment, or date of last scan).

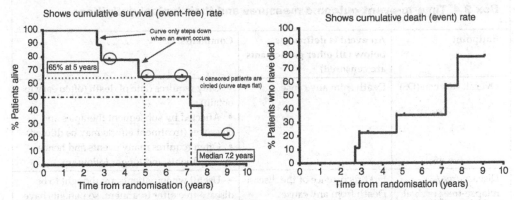

Figure 2.3 Kaplan–Meier plot of the survival data for nine patients, which can be used to estimate survival rates (vertical line drawn at 5 years) and median survival (horizontal line drawn at 50%) (left side). The reverse plot (right side) shows 100 minus the fourth column in Table 2.2.

interventions (called **non-informative censoring**), so that the risk of an event is expected to be similar between those who are censored and those still followed up. There may be concerns over:

- Too many censored participants (unless the event rate is naturally low)
- Too much censoring early on (i.e. not enough follow-up)
- Clear difference in censoring between trials arms being compared
- Censoring is associated with the trial treatment (e.g. patient stops trial treatment early due to a side effect, and they are censored at that date). This is called **informative censoring**, and it is problematic especially if this leads to unequal censoring between trial arms.[9]

With longer follow-up, someone initially censored at 3 years could then appear at 5 years.

We can now obtain summary statistics from the Kaplan–Meier plot. These are the **survival rate (proportion)** at a specific time point, and the **median survival; Figure 2.3**.

When all participants have had the event of interest, the Kaplan–Meier median survival is identical to the simple median seen from a ranked list of numbers. The median only tends to be different when participants are censored. Therefore, although the median is *calculated* in quite different ways when using either continuous or time-to-event measures, the *interpretation* of the median is practically the same. The median is used instead of the mean because time-to-event data often has a skewed distribution.

Many Kaplan–Meier plots start at 100% at time zero, i.e. the percentage of people *without* the event of interest (Figure 2.3, left side). This is useful when events tend to occur early on or there are many events. This can be reversed to start at 0% at time zero, i.e. the percentage of people *with* the event of interest (Figure 2.3, right side). This plot may be more informative when events tend to occur later on or the event rate is low because the upper limit of the y-axis can be less than 100%, allowing differences between two treatments to be seen more clearly. However, the y-axis scale is sometimes too small, making treatment differences seem larger than they actually are.

Different types of time-to-event measures

Box 2.4 shows commonly used time-to-event endpoints, and Figure 2.4 illustrates some of these. The event should always be clearly defined.

Box 2.4 Time-to-event outcome measures and their typical definitions

Endpoint	An event is defined as below (all other participants are censored)	Comments
Overall survival (OS)	Death from any cause	• Only requires date of death (often easy to obtain) • Affected by subsequent therapies and crossover (treatment effects may be diluted) • Often requires many events and hence many patients and longer follow-up
Disease-free/relapse-free survival (DFS/RFS)	First recurrence of the disease Death from any cause	• Useful when patients are thought to be disease-free after treatment, so patients have a good prognosis • Needs accurate date of recurrence/relapse • Not affected by subsequent therapies
Event-free survival (EFS)	First recurrence of the disease First occurrence of other specified diseases Death from any cause	
Progression-free survival (PFS) Duration of response (DOR)* Duration of clinical benefit (DCB)*	First sign of disease progression Death from any cause	• Useful for advanced diseases, where patients have not been 'cured' after treatment and are expected to deteriorate in the near future • Needs accurate date of progression • Not affected by subsequent therapies
Disease (or cause)-specific survival	Death from the disease of interest	• Needs accurate confirmation of cause of death (may not be reliably recorded) • Deaths from causes other than that of interest are not counted as an event (so could overestimate the overall benefit)
Time to treatment failure (TTF)	First sign of disease progression Death from any cause Stopped treatment	• Reflects changes in patient management (hence clinically relevant) • Reasons for stopping or starting new treatments may be heterogenous and not well recorded
Time to next treatment (TTNT)	Start of a new treatment for the disorder Death from any cause	
Time to remission	First sign of (positive) response or disease remission	• Can reflect fast-acting therapies
Treatment free interval (TFI)	Starting a later therapy (TFI is the time between this and the end of the previous therapy)	• Reflects changes in patient management

Recurrence: no clinical evidence of the disease shortly after treatment, but the disease returned later on.

Progression (or relapse): the person still had the disease after treatment, but it got worse later.

Disease and event-free survival may be used interchangeably, so be clear about the precise definition.

* Time starts from when the patient is in remission or responds and so only applies to these patients (unlike the other endpoints that usually start from the date of randomisation/registration and therefore based on all patients). DOR is often for patients who achieve CR or PR; DCB for patients who achieve CR, PR or SD.

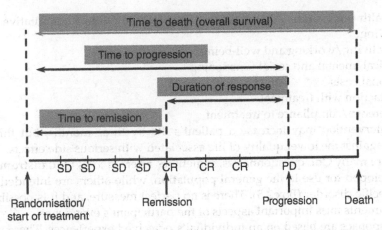

Figure 2.4 Illustration of some time-to-event outcome measures. CR complete remission/response; PD progressive disease (could also be recurrence/relapse); SD stable disease.

Even though labels such as OS and DFS imply something positive, we often focus on the events (i.e. we talk about the risk of dying or risk of disease occurrence). The number of events is usually more important than the number of trial participants (hence observing many events produces reliable results).

When an event is disease incidence,[#] recurrence or progression, the date is usually when the disease was first clinically diagnosed rather than when it occurred biologically. This date is usually when the person has one of the regular examinations specified in the trial protocol, or after they developed symptoms and received clinical confirmation. Participants in the trial arms should therefore have their regular examinations at a similar time to avoid a biased endpoint.

When the measure is based on two or more event types (called composite outcomes, see page 110) and a participant has both events, such as disease occurrence followed by death, it is usual to consider only the date of the first event in the analysis. This is because the patient may be managed differently afterwards: the trial treatment changes or stops, non-trial therapies are given or patients may be given the treatment from the other trial arm. It may then be difficult to attribute differences in the endpoint to the initial trial treatments.

2.7 Patient-reported outcome measures (PROMs)

Many trial endpoints are measured on participants by health professionals, i.e. clinical assessment and measures in biospecimens or from imaging scans. PROMs are outcome measures that come directly from the participant, of which **health-related quality of life (QoL)** is the most common. Most PROMs are obtained through self-completed questionnaires, completed by the trial participant, guardian or relative, or during an interview

---

[#] The first time the person develops the disease of interest.

with a health professional. The questionnaires aim to provide a quantitative measure of the following:

- Daily living/working and well-being
- Physical, mental and social functioning
- Personal costs
- Satisfaction with treatment
- Adherence/compliance to treatment

A new intervention may increase a patient's life by three months, but this could be balanced against the lower quality of life associated with serious side effects.

There are many QoL questionnaires, sometimes referred to as **QoL instruments**. Some were developed for use in the general population, while others are intended for people with a specific disorder (Box 2.5). There is no perfect measure, and it is possible that certain instruments miss important aspects of the participant's experience.

QoL responses are based on an individual's perceived experiences. These perceptions will vary between people and also over time within the same person.

When choosing a QoL instrument for a trial, it is necessary to determine whether it will measure what participants would consider important in that trial and whether it is sensitive enough to detect changes in QoL. If many participants report a very low (or very high) QoL score at baseline, there is not much scope to get a lower (or higher) score after treatment, called a floor (or ceiling) effect.

A **validated** QoL instrument is one that has been assessed and judged to measure what it is supposed to measure. The following questions are typical in making this judgement:

- Are the self-reported scores highly correlated with relevant objective or clinical outcomes? For example, if patients report high pain scores, do they also request, or use, more pain relief medication?
- Do the scores from a QoL instrument correlate with scores from another, perhaps well-established instrument, both of which aim to measure similar aspects of QoL?

Box 2.5 Examples of QoL instruments used in clinical trials

General population

- Short Form 12 or 36 (SF-12 or SF-36)
- General Health Questionnaire (GHQ-30)

Disease-specific

- European Organisation for Research and Treatment of Cancer (EORTC) QLQ C-30 (all cancer patients) and cancer-specific modules
- Functional Assessment of Cancer Therapy (FACT) and cancer-specific modules
- Parkinson's Disease Questionnaire
- Dermatology Life Quality Index (DLQI)
- Stroke and Aphasia Quality of Life Scale (SAQOL-39)

Psychological

- Hamilton Anxiety Scale (HAS)
- Hospital and Anxiety Depression Scale (HADS)
- Beck Depression Inventory (BDI).

Reliability can be assessed by judging whether a QoL instrument will produce similar scores when repeated in similar groups of people.

Participants usually rate their experiences or feelings for specific questions on the questionnaire, on an ordinal scale; e.g. none, a little, some, a lot (which is a form of categorical data/'counting people' endpoints). Each category is assigned a numerical score, and in the simplest situation, the total score for a person is obtained by summing scores across all questions. This total score usually looks like continuous data which can be analysed in the same way as in Section 2.5.

2.8 Summary points

- Trials should have clearly defined outcome measures (endpoints).
- Surrogate endpoints should be closely correlated with true/hard endpoints, and have been validated, especially if they are used as the main trial endpoint.
- Outcome measures could involve 'counting people', 'taking measurements on people' or 'time-to-event' data.
- Counting people: data are summarised by a percentage or proportion (risk).
- Taking measurements on people: data are summarised by average and spread (mean and standard deviation if the data are Normally distributed, median and interquartile range if the data are skewed).
- Time-to-event data: data can be summarised using a Kaplan–Meier plot, median value, or survival or event-rate at a specific time point.

References

1. Buyse M, Sargent DJ, Grothey A *et al.* Biomarkers and surrogate end points—the challenge of statistical validation. *Nat Rev Clin Oncol* 2010; **7**(6):309.
2. Aronson JK, Ferner RE. Biomarkers-A general review. *Curr Protoc Pharmacol* 2017; 76:9.23.1–9.23.17. doi: https://doi.org/10.1002/cpph.19.
3. Weintraub WS, Lüscher TF, Pocock S. The perils of surrogate endpoints. *Eur Heart J* 2015; **36**(33):2212–2218.
4. Guidance for industry: clinical trial endpoints for the approval of cancer drugs and biologics. https://www.fda.gov/media/71195/download.
5. Budd Haeberlein S, Aisen PS, Barkhof F *et al.* Two randomized phase 3 studies of Aducanumab in early Alzheimer's disease. *J Prev Alzheimers Dis* 2022; **9**(2):197–210.
6. Kirkwood B, Sterne J. *Essential Medical Statistics*. 2nd edn, Wiley-Blackwell, 2003.
7. Petrie A, Sabin C. *Medical Statistics at a Glance*. 4th edn, Wiley-Blackwell 2019.
8. Kaplan EL, Meier P. Nonparametric estimation from incomplete observations. *J Am Stat Assoc* 1958; **53**:457–481.
9. Templeton AJ, Amir E, Tannock IF. Informative censoring – a neglected cause of bias in oncology trials. *Nat Rev Clin Oncol* 2020; **17**(6):327–328.

CHAPTER 3

Phase I trials

Phase I trials are conducted to examine the biological and pharmacological actions of a new treatment (usually a drug) and its side effects. They are usually preceded by several laboratory studies: *in vitro* (using human biological samples) and those involving mammals. More details about the design, conduct and analysis of phase I trials are found in published reviews and guidance reports.[1-6]

3.1 Trial objectives

The most common objective is to find a dose (e.g. of a drug or radiotherapy) that is considered sufficiently safe but with some evidence of efficacy (activity) to warrant further studies, called a **dose-escalation trial**.

Phase I studies can also examine the pharmacological effects of an experimental drug according to sex, taking it with or without food, time of day, giving it as a single tablet per day or several tablets per day each with a smaller dose, examine whether it interacts with other medicines (drug-drug interactions), or determine frequency (e.g. whether to take the therapy every 1, 3 or 5 days). First-in-human phase I trials are when an experimental therapy is first administered to humans after laboratory and animal studies. The following are typically investigated in phase I trials (not always first-in-human studies):

- A new drug (unlicensed) to be used on its own (monotherapy) or combined with standard therapies, or a new medical device
- Drug is already licensed for an indication (disorder) and used in clinical practice, and the aim is to use it for a new indication
- Two licensed drugs for an indication to be combined for the first time for the same or other indication
- New form of radiotherapy or medical device

Phase I trials are meant to be relatively small and quick to conduct, but this is not often the case. Therefore, it is worth considering alternatives to stand alone phase I studies:

- Merge with a phase II trial (Chapter 4): Use a single protocol with a **Phase I/II** design. The regulatory authority and ethics board can review the protocol but give approval to only conduct the phase I stage first. After that has finished, the investigators submit the phase I findings with a recommended dose for phase II, before obtaining approval for that part of the protocol.
- **Safety run-in study** as part of a phase II or III trial: If there is already evidence on the drug or combination therapy being investigated (e.g. in another disorder or indication), and the purpose is only to confirm safety for a pre-specified dose of a new drug, it is

A Concise Guide to Clinical Trials, Second Edition. Allan Hackshaw.
© 2024 John Wiley & Sons Ltd. Published 2024 by John Wiley & Sons Ltd.

possible to design a phase II or III trial, but in the protocol specify a 'run-in' cohort. This involves recruiting a few patients first, typically 5–10, who receive the experimental therapy, and if there are no safety concerns, the trial proceeds to the next stage (phase II or III).

3.2 Types of participants

For many studies healthy volunteers are used initially, and if the experimental treatment is safe enough, there could follow other phase I trials of patients affected with the disorder of interest. An exception is cancer trials, where anti-cancer drugs or forms of radiotherapy are first tested in cancer patients because the expected toxic effects make them inappropriate to test in healthy volunteers. Furthermore, healthy people may be able to tolerate cancer drugs at higher doses than a cancer patient, who is already ill. Several phase I trials are based on patients who have had several previous therapies but did not respond, so they tend to have a poorer prognosis than the target group of patients (e.g. cancer). Therefore, estimates of treatment effectiveness need to be interpreted carefully. Investigators should therefore consider whether modern phase I studies should aim for patient populations that are more representative of the target for the experimental therapy.

3.3 Outcome measures

Many outcome measures are examined.

Adverse events (toxicities)

Adverse events can be minor (i.e. transient, not of material concern to the person taking the drug, and does not require any treatment) or major (clinically significant, impacts the person's daily living, and may require treatment and occasionally hospitalisation).

Many dose finding trials involve identifying a **dose-limiting toxicity (DLT)** which is integral to the study design (Box 3.1). DLTs need to be pre-defined in the trial protocol, and clearly specified so that treating clinicians and research staff can identify and record them reliably.

The principle aim is to find the **maximum tolerated dose (MTD)**. Sometimes, it is the dose at which a pre-specified number of individuals suffer a severe adverse event, indicating that this dose may be too unsafe, so the next lowest dose would be investigated further. This definition can also be called the **maximum administered dose**.

Box 3.1 Dose limiting toxicities (DLTs)

- DLTs are adverse events (reactions) considered to be causally related to the experimental drug(s) or medical device and unacceptable.
- They are often high grade symptoms and may require treatment, hospitalisation or early stopping of the experimental therapy (for chronic disorders some low grade toxicities may be unacceptable).
- They typically occur soon after drug administration (e.g. within 28 days).
- Investigators should try to distinguish a causally related toxicity from disease progression, expected adverse symptoms due to the disorder being treated, or natural progression of pre-existing medical conditions (e.g. someone who developed a myocardial infarction during the trial may have prior hypertension and abnormal lipid levels).

At other times, the MTD could be the dose that has an acceptable number of side effects and is therefore used in further studies.

Pharmacological endpoints

Pharmacological effects cover metabolism and excretion:

- **Pharmacodynamics (PD)**: physical or biological measures that show *how the drug affects the body*, including vital signs, blood pressure, body temperature, heart and respiratory rates, liver and renal function, and cardiac tests. PD measures might also represent biomarkers of activity assessed using imaging or molecular changes (e.g. plasma glucose for drugs for diabetes, or tumour target inhibition or activation for cancer). Toxicities can perhaps be considered an example of pharmacodynamics.
- **Pharmacokinetics (PK)**: physical or biological measures that show *how the body deals with the drug*, including drug uptake (absorption), distribution, metabolism, and excretion/elimination (Box 3.2).

Many endpoints are measured at multiple time points for each participant, the regularity of which depends on how quickly these effects are expected to be seen (e.g. could be every 2 hours or once every day). A plasma concentration-time curve is obtained for each participant (Figure 3.1), from which several pharmacokinetic parameters are calculated.

Box 3.2 Commonly used pharmacokinetic outcome measures

- **AUC (area under the curve):** indicates total drug exposure, using a plasma concentration–time curve (Figure 3.1).
- **Cmax:** the highest concentration level.
- **Tmax:** the time at which Cmax occurs.
- **Terminal half-life ($t_{1/2}$):** the time it takes for the plasma concentration to decrease by 50% in the final part of the curve, when the drug is being eliminated (here, the curve may appear as a straight line if using a log transformation of the plasma levels).
- **Clearance (CL):** the rate at which the drug is removed from the plasma as it is metabolised or excreted (CL = dose/AUC).
- **Volume of distribution (V):** the amount of drug in the body divided by the plasma concentration.
- **Bioavailability (F):** the percentage of administered dose that gets into the systemic circulation (an intravenous drug should have $F = 100\%$).

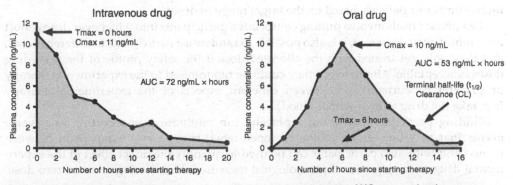

Figure 3.1   Plasma concentration-time curves for two trial participants. AUC area under the curve.

Efficacy endpoints

Standard efficacy outcome measures are often measured, acknowledging the small study size. Markers of treatment response including surrogate endpoints are typically used because they can be measured early. Biospecimens taken at baseline and during treatment could also be used for translational research, including genetic sequencing of samples, to see whether there are markers that differentiate responders and non-responders to the treatment.

As new safer therapies are developed, biological efficacy endpoints or pharmacological markers of drug activity become as important as toxicities. Vaccines, for example, have few expected side effects, and major toxicities are rare or unexpected. The objective could then be to find the *lowest* dose that has a clinically important effect on a biological marker of efficacy. This is in contrast to the MTD which is the *highest* tolerable dose, determined using pre-specified toxicities. The lowest effective dose can be referred to as the **minimum biologically active dose, minimum effective dose (MED) or optimum biological dose**. This dose is determined using endpoints that measure biological activity or efficacy response. Toxicity is still monitored closely, but the efficacy indicators have a higher weight when determining which dose is carried forward to a phase II study. The MTD and MED could be very different in which case the chosen dose for further study might depend on costs and safety.

The Food and Drug Administration (FDA) Oncology Center of Excellence has established Project Optimus that encourages investigators to explore and generate more evidence on the optimum schedule (dose, treatment frequency or duration) during drug development before new therapies are launched.[7] This is because a similar efficacy can sometimes be achieved with a lower dose or shorter duration but with the benefits of improved patient tolerability, fewer adverse events and better health-related quality of life.[7,8] The cost of drugs would also be cheaper, which is a major consideration for low and middle income countries. Instead of using phase I studies to select a single dose (or regimen) to take forwards to phase II or III, two or more doses should be evaluated, ideally in a randomised trial, using markers of efficacy. The Methodology for the Development of Innovative Cancer Therapies (MDICT) Taskforce provides practical guidance on this.[9]

3.4 Designs

There is a wide variety of phase I designs. The basic premise of a dose-escalation study is to give a certain dose to a few participants (referred to as a dose cohort or dose group), and if tolerable, the next group receive a higher dose. This continues until the MTD is found.

The total number of participants recruited will depend on the design employed and how many doses are evaluated. The trial protocol could specify what might be a maximum number of patients, based on the target range of doses.

Most phase I trials involve putting consecutive participants into whichever dose cohort is currently open. However, it is also possible to **randomise** participants to different doses, and they only get treated with the allocated dose if the safety profile of the preceding doses is acceptable. Alternatively, they could be randomised to the experimental therapy or **placebo** concurrently, or between different aspects of the experimental therapy (e.g. take the drug with or without food).

Blinding participants by using a **placebo** can minimise over-reporting of adverse events that may be seen in unblinded (open label) trials, and a comparison between treated and untreated participants can be used to quantify the direct effect of the experimental drug on biological and physiological measures. Also, having a 'no or zero dose' group acts an anchor when modelling the relationship between toxicities (DLTs) and dose. However, the effort and costs of manufacturing placebos, the randomisation process and other trial conduct procedures required for a blinded trial may not be worthwhile in all situations.

Some phase I trials involve **intrapatient dose escalation**, whereby the dose is incrementally increased in the *same* participant. This is usually in studies of people who already have the disorder of interest, and the potential advantage is that the chance of obtaining benefit can be maximised by tolerating a higher dose. However, toxicities can take time to accumulate, so it might be difficult to ascertain a MTD when each patient has had several different doses.

Phase 0 trials are a special case of a phase I trial, and specifically for first-in-human studies. They are based on a few patients (<10), and the dose given is typically so small that it is unlikely to have any material impact on the disorder or lead to symptomatic side effects. The primary intention is not to examine the relationship between drug dose and toxicity but rather whether the drug can reach the target tissue or organs and how the body deals with the drug. Patients are usually monitored closely using scans and blood samples.

Phase I designs are either rule-based or model-based, and they each have their strengths and limitations (Box 3.3).

Box 3.3 Features of dose-escalation trial designs

Rule-based	Model-based
A+B designs often used.	Continual reassessment method often used.
Assumes nothing about the shape of relationship between dose and risk of DLT.	A mathematical relationship between dose and DLT risk is assumed (flattened S-shaped curve).*
Easy to understand and implement (can be done by hand).	Requires expertise in Bayesian statistics and specialist software.
Assessment of a dose cohort ignores other doses.	Assessment uses all dose cohorts.
Assessment done after each cohort has been treated.	Model is updated in real time to determine the dose for the next patient.
If many lower dose cohorts have no DLTs, it can take a long time and many patients to reach the MTD.	Can skip lower doses that have no DLTs or have only 1 patient per dose; so quicker to reach the MTD.
Three to six patients are often enough to examine the pharmacological actions of the drug.	A dose cohort of only one patient might yield insufficient information about response and the pharmacological actions of the therapy.
Cannot easily handle two or more factors changing at the same time.	Can evaluate two factors simultaneously (e.g. doses of two experimental drugs or two drugs one with varying dose and the other with varying frequency of administration).

*Using for example Bayesian models or maximum likelihood methods.

Rule-based designs

For many years, **rule-based designs** were the most commonly used, and still are but to a lesser extent.

A+B designs (A and B each represents a number of people) involve recruiting 'A' participants first and if needed 'B' participants are enrolled to the same dose cohort. They assume a certain DLT rate, above which is considered unacceptable. The most popular has been the **3+3 design** (Figure 3.2), where the DLT rate is assumed to be 33%. Although such designs are simple to use they can be inefficient.

One design that attempts to mitigate some of the issues over the 3+3 design is called an **accelerated titration design** (Figure 3.3). A key feature is that the first few dose cohorts

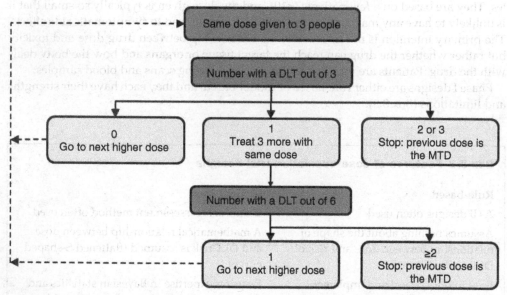

Figure 3.2 Flowchart for a phase I trial using a '3+3' design. MTD (maximum tolerated dose); DLT (dose-limiting toxicity). Doses are increased until the maximum planned dose or MTD is reached.

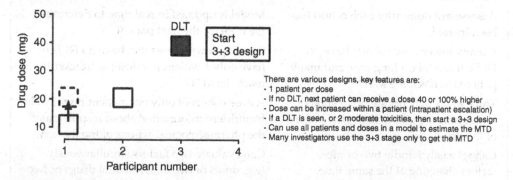

Figure 3.3 Accelerated titration design (open square indicates no DLT; solid square indicates that the participant experienced a DLT). Because participant 3 had a DLT, participant 4 would be enrolled into a traditional 3+3 design, with two other people. The open dashed square for participant 1 represents a dose increase for this person.

each contain only one participant, hence the term 'accelerated', so should be quicker to run than a 3+3 approach.

Although model-based designs (next section) are increasingly used, if there are only 2 or 3 planned doses, a standard A+B (e.g. 3+3) design should be acceptable, with little or no gain in having a more complex model-based method. Software for A+B designs are fairly easy to use and freely available.[10]

Model-based designs

Model-based designs are considered to be more efficient than rule-based designs, though this is not always guaranteed. Funding organisations are now familiar with these approaches, so may expect investigators to consider them in grant applications.

A commonly used design is the **continual reassessment method (CRM)**.[11] Investigators specify the initial relationship (using guesses of the numerical parameters of the model) and then, after each participant has been given the therapy and assessed, the shape and/or position of the curve is changed using regression analyses; Figure 3.4. There are modified versions of the CRM; the **escalation with overdose control** (EWOC) which uses modelling to minimise the chance that a participant will be given a dose with an unacceptable DLT rate; and the **time-to-event continual reassessment method** (TITE-CRM) which accounts for exposure time to the experimental therapy and is therefore suitable when toxicities may occur sometime after treatment has started (e.g. radiotherapy).

Dose de-escalation designs

Most trials start with the lowest dose, and then successive participant cohorts receive higher doses. However, there are situations where the investigators already have sufficient

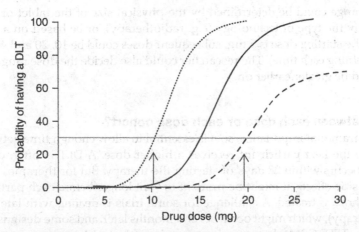

Figure 3.4 Continual reassessment method. The solid (middle) curve is the initial curve before patients are treated, using guesses (estimates) of the DLT rate at each dose. A DLT rate of >30% is considered unacceptable (horizontal line). If the starting dose is 15 mg and there is no DLT, a re-modelled curve (large dashes; right curve) indicates that the next dose could be 20 mg. If there is a DLT using 15 mg, the re-modelled curve (small dashes) indicates 10 mg as the next dose because the expected DLT rate is <30% in both cases (the arrows).

prior information about the safety profile of a new therapy and so wish to start off with what they think is the MTD. Typically, 3–6 participants could be recruited at this dose, and if there are no DLTs the trial stops, or a further 3–6 participants might be enrolled to confirm the safety profile. If there are DLTs, successive cohorts receive lower doses, and a rule- or model-based design can be employed.

Dose de-escalation trials represent a quick and relatively inexpensive approach. The main issue is the potential for harm by exposing participants to a high dose level. If there is uncertainty over dose and toxicities, it might be more prudent to have a standard dose escalation approach.

Which doses?

The starting dose for many first-in-man trials is based on animal experiments. Different countries have their own regulatory requirements. For example, the US Food and Drug Administration require evidence from mammalian species. The starting dose could be 1/10th down to 1/100th of the NOAEL (No Observable Adverse Effect Level: the highest dose that does not lead to toxicities in the most sensitive animal species).

For other phase I trials, there are several methods for determining the dose range. If a therapy is already in use, the starting dose could be the same dose currently used, or if there is concern over toxicity a lower dose is chosen, particularly if it will be combined with another therapy. Laboratory (*in vitro*) studies could be used to justify the starting dose. Some investigators use a Fibonacci sequence. The series starts off with '1', and then every successive number is the sum of the preceding two numbers. The first 5 numbers in the series are 1, 2, 3, 5 and 8. The relative increase between adjacent doses is roughly constant (almost two-thirds, e.g. $8/5 = 1.6$). If the starting dose of an oral drug is 3 mg, the dose cohorts would be 3, 6, 9, 15 and 24 mg, which could be rounded ('modified Fibonacci' sequence).

The dose range could be determined by the physical size of the tablet or capsule, be constrained by the type of technology (e.g. radiotherapy), or be based on a logarithmic scale (e.g. if the starting dose is 5 mg, subsequent doses could be 10, 20 and 40 mg, representing a doubling each time). The researcher could also decide the dose range, where the increase could be greater earlier on.

How long between each dose or each dose cohort?

Safety is of paramount importance, so it is essential to allow enough time between a dose cohort before the next participant receives a higher dose. A DLT is often defined as a toxicity that occurs within 28 days of starting the therapy. But for therapies expected to have serious side effects, it might be prudent to wait longer before each participant, and each dose cohort, is treated. A challenge for some trials is dealing with late side effects (e.g. radiotherapy), which might occur several months later, and some designs can handle with this (e.g. TITE-CRM). In some situations, investigators have to accept time delays between dose cohorts.

Although the DLT time period is pre-specified in the protocol (e.g. 28 days, or in cancer trials the first 1 or 2 cycles of chemotherapy), adverse events should still be collected afterwards for all participants. Occasionally, the accumulated adverse events will influence the choice of the MTD, not just those defined as a DLT.

3.5 Conducting the trial

Trial participants must be monitored closely, and this is usually done by admitting them to a special clinical trials facility, allowing regular investigations over 24 hours or longer, such as blood tests and physical examinations. If there is already evidence on the drug's safety profile, participants may be seen as outpatients, but they still need to be examined regularly (e.g. at least once a week). Participants are often found through advertisements in the media, and those accepted onto a trial programme are paid for taking part (usually for commercial company trials). For trials of people who already have the disorder of interest, their treating clinician would approach them for the study.

If the drug, medical device or radiotherapy technique has not been previously tested in humans, the protocol needs to be followed very carefully to avoid unnecessary harm without protocol deviations or violations. Some phase I trials are considered 'high risk' by regulatory authorities and therefore more likely to be inspected.

Pre-specifying what constitutes a DLT can be difficult even when done by experts. Sometimes the definitions result in too many patients being classified as having a DLT, and then the trial cannot proceed to higher (more effective) doses. If this happens, it might be best to suspend the trial and re-examine the DLT definitions, then re-start the study with a revised list of events that has been reviewed by independent experts.

Once the MTD has been determined, it is good practice to test the dose on a further group of, say, 5–10 participants, to obtain a clearer view of the safety profile, and perhaps efficacy, before proceeding to a larger study.

3.6 Statistical analysis and reporting the trial results

Phase I trials are usually straightforward to analyse and write up. They consist of:
- A summary of the patient and disease characteristics.
- A summary of adverse events (including severity).
- A clear outline (preferably as a table) showing exactly how the MTD was obtained, by listing each DLT at every dose, what they were and the severity grade.
- Treatment-related deaths should be described in detail.
- A summary of adherence to the experimental therapy, including how many patients stopped early and why.
- Summary statistics for the pharmacokinetic and pharmacodynamic measures (e.g. means and standard deviations). Outcomes such as the mean AUC might not be interpretable on their own, and are better used for comparing between doses. Showing that AUC increases proportionally with dose (i.e. AUC doubles as the dose doubles), makes it easier to describe and model the effect of the drug, and plan further early phase studies.

An example of a simple phase I trial with placebo is given in Box 3.4. Note that there were 5 doses so a model-based design probably would have been used if the trial was conducted now. Any evidence of efficacy/activity can also be reported, acknowledging the small number of patients limits the reliability of these analyses. This is usually done for each participant. Figure 3.5 is an example using cancer but it can be applied to other disorders, showing a waterfall plot of the change in tumour size before and after using the experimental therapy for each patient.

Box 3.4 Example of finding the MTD in a phase I trial. Source: Adapted from Wensing et al.[12]

Study feature	Example
Target disease	Parkinson's disease
Drug being investigated	BAY 63-9044, an 5-HT_{1a}-receptor agonist (has neuroprotective and symptomatic effects)
Aim	To determine the maximum tolerated dose
Design	First-in-man trial of male healthy volunteers, aged 18–45 years (randomised study)
Treatment doses investigated	0.25, 0.50, 1.20, 2.50, 5.00 mg and placebo
Definition of dose-limiting toxicity, DLT	Any adverse event considered drug-related (graded mild, moderate, severe)
Number of participants	$N = 45$
Main result	No serious adverse events
	Number of mild or moderate events out of the number of participants in the cohort were:
	Placebo $n = 0/14$
	0.25 mg $n = 2/7$
	0.50 mg $n = 0/7$
	1.20 mg $n = 0/6$
	2.50 mg $n = 1/5$
	5.00 mg $n = 5/6$
Conclusion	Too many participants had adverse events using 5 mg.
Maximum tolerated dose (MTD)	2.5 mg should be used in further studies.

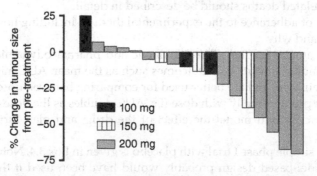

Figure 3.5 A waterfall plot showing, for each trial participant (each bar), the change in tumour size from baseline (pre-treatment) to after using the experimental therapy. The highest dose tended to have the most number of responders (i.e. they had a material reduction in tumour size).

3.7 Summary points

• Phase I studies should be small and aim to provide a first assessment of safety in human participants, or for new combinations of therapies, or application of a licensed therapy to a different disorder or indication.

• There are simple (rule-based) designs for determining the dose of a new therapy that has an acceptable number of side effects, but where several doses are examined model-based designs should be more efficient.

• Investigators can be flexible in their choice of design. Trials of new, safer therapies can have different biological endpoints as well as toxicity.

• Reports of phase I studies should provide clear information on the pharmacological properties of a new drug, including plasma concentration curves over time, and details of adverse events.

References

1. Eisenhauer EA, Twelves C, Buyse M. *Phase I Cancer Clinical Trials: A Practical Guide*. Oxford University Press, 2006.
2. Le Tourneau C, Lee JJ, Siu LL. Dose escalation methods in phase I cancer clinical trials. J Natl Cancer Inst 2009; **101**(10):708–720.
3. Cook N, Hansen AR, Siu LL, Abdul Razak AR. Early phase clinical trials to identify optimal dosing and safety. Mol Oncol 2015; **9**(5):997–1007.
4. Guideline on strategies to identify and mitigate risks for first-in-human and early clinical trials with investigational medicinal products. European Medicines Agency. EMEA/CHMP/SWP/28367/07 Rev. 1. Committee for Medicinal Products for Human Use (CHMP) 2017.
5. Guidelines for Phase I clinical trials. Association of the British Pharmaceutical Industry (ABPI) 2018.
6. Center for Drug Evaluation and Research (CDER). Content and format of Investigational New Drug Applications (INDs) for Phase 1 Studies of Drugs, Including Well-Characterized, Therapeutic, Biotechnology-derived Products. CfBEaRC. 1995. https://www.fda.gov/regulatory-information/search-fda-guidance-documents/contentand-format-investigational-new-drug-applications-inds-phase-1-studies-drugs-including-well.
7. Food and Drug Administration, Project Optimus. https://www.fda.gov/about-fda/oncology-center-excellence/project-optimus.
8. Shah M, Rahman A, Theoret MR, Pazdur R. The drug-dosing conundrum in oncology-when less is more. N Engl J Med. 2021;385:1445–1447.
9. Araujo D, Greystoke A, Bates S, *et al*. Oncology phase I trial design and conduct: time for a change - MDICT Guidelines 2022. Ann Oncol. 2023;34(1):48–60.
10. Wheeler GM, Sweeting MJ, Mander AP. Aplus B: a web application for investigating A + B designs for phase I cancer clinical trials. PLoS One 2016; **11**(7):e0159026.
11. Wheeler GM, Mander AP, Bedding A *et al*. How to design a dose-finding study using the continual reassessment method. BMC Med Res Methodol 2019; **19**(1):18.
12. Wensing G, Haase C, Brendel E, Bottcher MF. Pupillography as a sensitive, non-invasive biomarker in healthy volunteers: first-in-man study of BAY 63-9044, a new 5-HT$_{1a}$-receptor agonist with dopamine agnostic properties. *Eur J Clin Pharmacol* 2007; **63**:1123–1128.

CHAPTER 4

Phase II trials

Key design features of phase II studies are covered in Chapter 1, and there are elements from Chapter 5 that can also apply to randomised phase II studies.

4.1 Trial objectives

The aim of many phase II studies is to obtain *preliminary* evidence on whether a new treatment might be effective, used to justify and inform the design of a subsequent phase III trial. However, some phase II trials can change clinical practice directly, usually for rare disorders (where it is unfeasible to conduct a large phase III study), where there is a clear unmet need (no improvement over standard of care for many years), or for diseases with very poor prognoses, are life-threatening or are severely debilitating.

A major problem with drug development and other types of interventions is that many phase III trials 'fail', i.e. they do not show the expected benefit. Sometimes this is due to investigators who have taken a gamble by conducting a large confirmatory study without sufficient prior evidence. Other times, the preceding phase II studies have had inadequate designs, unrealistic assumptions about the treatment effect, or they included participants who were unrepresentative of those examined in a phase III study. Better phase II designs should lower the phase III trial 'failure' rate.

4.2 Designs

There is no single definition of what makes a trial 'phase II' and also to contrast it from phase III, but the following features can be used:
- Feasibility study to assess recruitment or ability to deliver an intervention
- Single-arm study without a comparator (control) therapy
- Main outcome measure is a surrogate marker.
- Sample size uses statistical significance tests that are one-sided and more than 5%, and occasionally power could be <80% (see Section 4.4).

Pilot or feasibility studies

Phase II studies may be **pilot** or **feasibility studies** used to assess whether a large phase III trial is likely to be successful. They could stand alone or be designed and conducted in a similar manner to a phase III trial (Chapter 5), but the protocol specifies that an early assessment is made after a proportion of participants have been recruited first (e.g. 25%) or the trial has run for a fixed length of time. This usually examines the proportion of

A Concise Guide to Clinical Trials, Second Edition. Allan Hackshaw.
© 2024 John Wiley & Sons Ltd. Published 2024 by John Wiley & Sons Ltd.

eligible participants approached who agree to enrol (i.e. the **acceptance** or **uptake rate**), and if accrual is low, what might be the likely reasons for this, and how to fix the problem. A formal sample size calculation for this part of the study is not normally necessary.

Designs for examining efficacy and safety

There are many phase II designs[1-3]; Figure 4.1. Most approaches are used to determine whether a new intervention is likely to be better than current treatments, based on an improvement in disease status or symptoms, or fewer side effects. Having several designs to choose from allows flexibility, to take into account feasibility and financial costs, as well as the scientific goals. Sample sizes are easily obtained using books or software, and more details are given in Section 4.4 (including definitions of statistical significance/error rate and power used below).[4-9]

Throughout this chapter, the terms 'response' and 'response rate' are used as generic labels for any health-related endpoint that indicates benefit for the participant, i.e. clinical efficacy, improvement in safety or biological activity.

Single-arm study

The simplest design has only one group, where all participants are given the experimental intervention. The advantage is that all resources, including financial costs, are concentrated on one group. Figure 4.2 is a typical design.

In the example in Figure 4.2, we need to see at least 13 responders out of 44 patients to justify further studies. This is 29.5% (13/44), which does not appear to match the target of 35%. However, the sample size is such that a lower one-sided 90% confidence interval (i.e. 10% statistical significance or error rate) exceeds 20%,[#] because this indicates that the

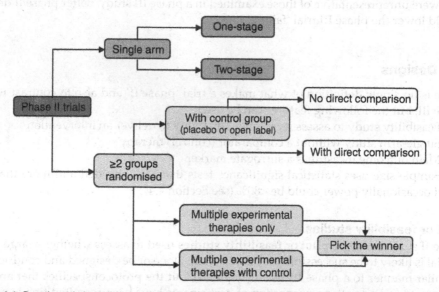

Figure 4.1 Overview of phase II trial designs. Single-arm trials are sometimes labelled as **phase IIa** and randomised trials as **phase IIb**. 'Direct comparison' means that the efficacy (or other) endpoints are pre-planned to be compared between the groups using statistical methods that produce a single effect size and p-value, and this is part of the design. Open label: where the trial interventions cannot be blinded.

[#] see section 4.4.

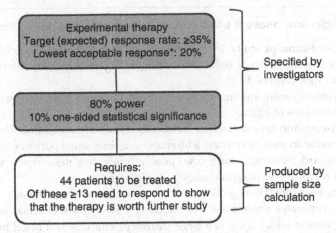

Figure 4.2 Typical outline of a single-arm phase II trial (power and statistical significance are explained later in the chapter). *could represent what is seen typically using current treatments.

possible **true** underlying response rate exceeds our lowest acceptable rate. This is enough evidence to consider further investigation of the therapy, particularly if other endpoints look favourable.

More complex designs can be used, including Bayesian approaches and methods that can deal with two primary outcome measures (e.g. response rate and toxicity).

Single-arm trials are appealing because of their simplicity. However, they are also one of the reasons why subsequent phase III trials fail to show a benefit. Integral to the design of many single-arm studies is the lowest acceptable response rate. This often comes from past studies of the standard treatment, considered to be the comparator for the experimental therapy, or simply personal experience from clinical practice. This is an example of **historical controls**. With advances in how patients are managed and the use of effective background therapies over time, the lowest acceptable response rate (controls) might be higher in current practice than historically. Investigators then over-estimate the effect of their experimental therapy when compared with historical controls.

Despite the concerns over single-arm studies, they still have some value (Box 4.1). They can also be compared with controls from real-world data using indirect comparisons (see Chapter 9). Nevertheless, it is always best to try to conduct a randomised phase II trial, even for uncommon disorders (though this may require national or international co-operation).

Single-arm two-stage study

In a two-stage design, the intervention is first tested on a small number of participants, who are assessed at the end of the first stage (Figure 4.3). The aim is to stop the trial early if the new therapy *appears* to be ineffective. Two-stage designs are useful when the new intervention might have serious side effects or is expensive, because only a few participants are initially given it, when it may have no true benefit. Some two-stage designs can incorporate both response and toxicity at the same time (e.g. Bryant and Day).[5]

After the first stage is reached, centres either suspend recruitment until the initial assessment is made or they continue recruiting patients. The latter is often done when the accrual rate is low, though the regulatory agency and ethics board may need to approve this.

Box 4.1 Single-arm phase II trials can be acceptable and scientifically useful

• As a **proof-of-concept study** in a relatively small number of participants, i.e. first assessment of activity/efficacy before launching a larger study particularly for a novel single agent or new class of drug
• Where the management and treatment of historical controls have been stable over time, particularly measures of efficacy
• For rare/uncommon disorders where randomised trials are unfeasible. This is especially relevant for precision medicine where a biomarker defines small patient subgroups
• Where standard treatments have low/poor efficacy, but the efficacy seen with the experimental therapy is striking and unexpectedly high
• The trial shows a (new) biological mechanism of action of a new therapy
• The trial incorporates a biomarker that validates a mechanism of action used to select a subset of patients in which there is a large treatment effect, or is a novel biomarker that shows how patients respond to the investigational therapy.

Adapted from Cannistra.[10]

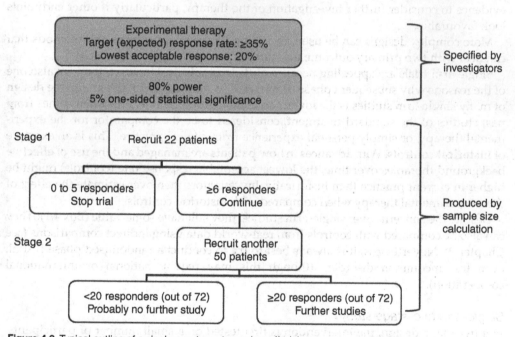

Figure 4.3 Typical outline of a single-arm two-stage phase II trial.

Randomised phase II trial with control arm

There are two trial groups: the new intervention and a control (which can be a standard of care therapy or placebo). This design has two fundamentally different approaches (Figure 4.4). One design is essentially a single-arm trial for the experimental therapy (Figure 4.4, left side), but in addition the investigators simply choose a certain number of control participants. Participants are randomised, but the primary efficacy analysis is the same as that for a single-arm study. A secondary analysis involving a direct statistical

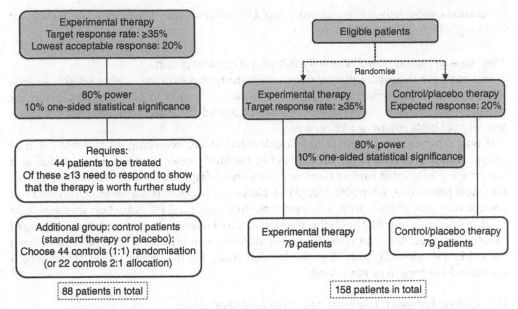

Figure 4.4 Typical outline of two types of randomised phase II trials with control arm (the number of participants and responders come from a sample size calculation). The left-hand side design does not involve a direct comparison of endpoints between the experimental and control therapy groups (it is essentially a single-arm study that happens to have a control group, and participants are randomised between them). The right-hand side design does involve a direct comparison.

comparison between the two groups (see Chapter 6) could be done, but the study was not designed for this. The control group is used to check that the estimate of the lowest acceptable response rate (e.g. using historical controls) is similar to the observed rate among controls now. If they are very different, interpreting the experimental group results could be problematic.

However, using the control group as a check only wastes information. It is better to have a direct statistical comparison between the experimental and control groups. This design (Figure 4.4, right side) is very similar to a randomised phase III trial, and indeed the statistical analyses are the same in that they produce a single effect size (Chapter 6). The key difference between this form of randomised phase II study and a phase III trial is that several design parameters used for the sample size calculation are relaxed.

A randomised phase II trial might be viewed as a quick and cheap randomised phase III trial, but it is not usually designed to provide definitive evidence on efficacy. This is reflected in the smaller sample size of 158 participants (Figure 4.4). A corresponding phase III design (5% two-sided statistical significance, instead of 10% one-sided) would require 276 participants.

Using randomisation also provides information on recruitment rates, and willingness to participate in a larger randomised (phase III) study.

Investigators of drug trials sometimes consider whether the control group should have **placebo** (double-blind) or not (open-label). While using placebos might be essential for a potentially practice-changing phase III trial, the cost of producing, implementing and distributing them in a phase II study might outweigh the scientific benefits. However, if sufficient resources are available, using placebo would strengthen the results and conclusions, especially when outcomes could be influenced by the assessor or participant knowing which treatment was given.

The value of randomised phase II trials with a control group

A real example illustrates how a randomised study can provide a more reliable assessment than a single-arm trial (Box 4.2).[11] The objective was to evaluate nintedanib for patients with advanced ovarian cancer who had already finished standard chemotherapy and were at high risk of cancer relapse.

It was designed as a randomised double-blind study, requiring 40 patients per trial group. Had this been a single-arm trial only, the study objective would have failed and the drug not evaluated further because the observed response for nintedanib (16.3%) was far below the lowest acceptable rate (50%). However, 16.3% was higher than the observed control response (5.0%), with a hazard ratio indicating a 35% reduction in the risk of progressing or dying. Although the investigators had over-estimated the response rates at the design stage, the trial showed a clear difference in efficacy that would have been missed in a single-arm study. This randomised study led to a larger phase III trial which confirmed the benefit of nintedanib.

Randomised phase II trial with several intervention arms

Two or more experimental treatment regimens could be examined simultaneously, e.g. several doses or treatment durations of the same drug, or different therapies. Each group is designed as a single-arm study, and participants are randomised to the different groups. One or more of the new treatments are identified that could be investigated further. This design is sometimes called **pick the winner**, though there is not necessarily a single winner. Even though participants are randomised, the primary intention is not to directly compare the results between the experimental treatment arms. Deciding which treatment regimen should be taken further is determined in the same way as with a single-arm phase II study, i.e. whether the treatment response rate in each arm exceeds the expected response associated with standard treatments. The one with the highest response (numerically) is often chosen. However, other outcome measures, especially toxicity, will be considered when choosing which arm(s) are investigated further. This design could also include a control arm, thus allowing for direct comparisons with each of the experimental arms, and two-stage approaches can be employed.

Box 4.2 Example of a randomised phase II trial illustrating the value of a control arm. Source: Adapted from Ledermann et al.[11]

Trial arm	9-month progression-free survival rate	
	Expected, used in the design	Observed at the end of the trial
Nintedanib ($n = 43$)	70%	16.3%
Placebo (control) ($n = 40$)	50% (lowest acceptable rate)	5.0%
		Hazard ratio 0.65 ($p = 0.06$)

Biomarker-driven phase II trials

Biomarkers support the development of targeted therapies (personalised medicine) designed to benefit some but not all patients with a certain disorder. They can be measured at baseline and during the trial.

Examples of biomarker-directed trials are **basket trials** (one treatment for several disorders or several subtypes of a disorder that have some common biomarker) or **umbrella trials** (several treatments for one disorder subdivided according to different biomarkers)[12]; Figure 4.5. Umbrella trials can also be called **platform trials**. They represent an efficient way of evaluating multiple drugs or multiple disorders because there is a single trial protocol. Bayesian statistics and **adaptive designs** are well suited to these studies. Adaptive designs allow study size to change during the trial, or treatment arms to be dropped or new ones added.

An example of a basket trial involved identifying patients who had a specific BRAF-V600-positive tumour, where they could have one of several cancer types (e.g. lung, breast, multiple myeloma, ovarian and colorectal). They were all given the same drug vemurafenib.[13] They could all be analysed as a single group. However, a challenge for basket trials is trying to determine whether the experimental treatment is similarly effective across all disease types or subtypes when the number of patients is likely to be very small in some subtypes. Descriptive and Bayesian statistics may help, and several efficacy endpoints should be examined.

An example of an umbrella trial is plasmaMATCH, in which patients with advanced breast cancer were stratified into 5 categories based on molecular typing of their cancer using circulating tumour DNA: ESR1 (estrogen receptor gene 1) mutation, HER2 (human epidermal growth factor receptor2) mutation, AKT1 mutation with oestrogen receptor-positive cancer and AKT1 mutation with oestrogen receptor-negative cancer or *PTEN* mutation. Each of these groups received a specific targeted anti-cancer agent and efficacy was evaluated separately.[14]

Umbrella trial: one disorder – several drugs for several markers

Basket trial: several disease types (or subtypes) – one drug for the same marker

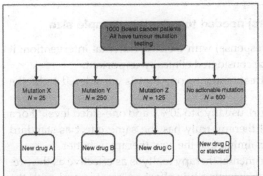
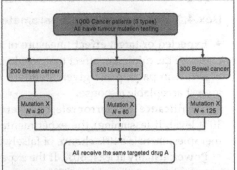

Figure 4.5 Outline of an umbrella and basket trial design. Adaptive randomisation could be used in umbrella designs where the first several (e.g. 50) patients are randomised using standard methods, and after an efficacy assessment is made, further patients are allocated to the drug that has the highest chance of response given the mutation status (using Bayesian methods). Randomisation to a control therapy (if used) is best done in *each* drug or disease subtype group but may be unfeasible with small groups.

Considerations for randomised umbrella designs include:
- Endpoints should be measured and analysed relatively quickly to adapt the randomisation allocation ratio in a timely fashion.
- The design is focussed on a single endpoint (measure of response); others should also be examined carefully for signs of efficacy/activity.

4.3 Outcome measures (see also Section 5.8, page 66)

There will be several outcome measures because sufficient information is needed to decide whether a larger phase III trial is justified. They will cover the key areas, especially efficacy and adverse events, though the value of collecting lots of quality of life (QoL) data in small trials is uncertain, especially single-arm studies. Sometimes, investigators might collect QoL just to see how it changes over time, to check that QoL is largely unaffected by the experimental therapy or to help design a larger study.

Surrogate efficacy endpoints are often used. Generally (but not always the case), a large effect on a surrogate endpoint is associated with a moderate/smaller effect on a true or hard endpoint.

4.4 Estimating study size

There are various methods for estimating how many participants should be recruited, which depend on the study design (single or two-stage, and randomised or not).

Several pieces of information are generally required (Box 4.3), which go into one of various statistical formulae to produce the sample size. There are free software, online/web calculators and commercial software.[4-9] Bayesian methods can also be used, with sample sizes produced from simulation studies (many hypothetical trials are created using the design parameters) rather than using a single formula.

The response (treatment effect) in the experimental and control arms can come from other similar studies, prior laboratory work or simply a good guess. It is bad practice to

---

Box 4.3 Information (input parameters) needed to calculate sample size

- **Expected or target effect** (measure of response) with the experimental intervention: it could be the minimum effect that would be considered clinically important.
- **Effect** in participants given **standard treatments**, or one that is considered to be the lowest acceptable response.
- **Significance level (error rate; type I error):** usually 5 to 20%,[3] and one-sided level.* For a 10% level, if (assuming) the experimental therapy truly has the same effect as standard therapies, there is a 10% chance of falsely claiming that the new therapy is better.
- **Power:** usually at least 80%. If the experimental therapy really is as effective as the pre-specified target, there is an 80% chance of detecting this effect or greater, and with the pre-specified significance level.

*Interest is only in the new therapy being better; for phase III trials we allow the new therapy to be better or worse hence two-sided levels are generally used.

Table 4.1 Sample size for phase II trials, where the response rate for controls (lowest acceptable response) is assumed to be 15%. The table shows the number of participants needed for the experimental treatment group.

One-sided statistical significance (80% power)	Target response rate for the experimental group (%)					
	Single-arm trial			Randomised trial: direct comparison with the controls		
	20	25	30	20	25	30
5%	360	101	48	714	197	95
10%	260	75	37	520	144	69
15%	207	62	29	407	113	54
20%	170	49	21	327	90	44

The single-arm trial can become a randomised phase II *without* direct comparison by randomly allocating the same number of participants as the experimental group to the control therapy (1:1 ratio) or half the number (2:1 ratio). In the randomised trial with direct comparison the same number of participants in the table is randomly allocated to the control group.

deliberately specify an overly large treatment effect just to make the sample size small, because such an effect would probably never occur so the trial can fail due to not reaching the target effect and statistical significance not being achieved.

Table 4.1 shows examples of sample sizes. Study size gets smaller as the expected treatment effect gets bigger (15 vs 20%, then 15 vs 30%), or by having higher values for statistical significance. Sample size also increases with increasing power.

Knowing that significance levels (error rates) can be higher than 5% allows investigators to consider feasibility of recruitment. Suppose an experimental therapy is expected to increase the response rate from 15% (standard therapy) to 25%. However, investigators can only recruit about 50–60 participants in a timely fashion. It would be a risky strategy to specify a treatment effect of 15 versus 30% just because this requires a study size of 48 participants (5% statistical significance). It is better to maintain the 15 versus 25%, but instead use a higher statistical significance of 15% (62 participants) or 20% (49 participants). The target effect is more likely to be achieved and is therefore viewed as a successful trial.

A single-arm phase II study will always be smaller (approximately half) than the experimental arm of a corresponding phase II trial with a direct comparison; Table 4.1 (e.g. 101 vs 197, and 48 vs 95). In single-arm trials, the sample size calculation assumes only one area of uncertainty, i.e. the new intervention arm, and that we know (with certainty) the effect using standard treatments. However, the sample size calculation for a randomised phase II study with a direct comparison assumes that the treatment effect in each arm is not known with certainty, i.e. *each* trial arm has imprecision when estimating efficacy, hence a larger sample size.

If the sample size for a randomised trial with a direct comparison is unlikely to be feasible, it is often better to have a randomised trial without a direct comparison (even 2:1 allocation ratio) rather than a single-arm study. Having a concurrent control group always provides useful information.

There are specific sample size methods for single-arm studies, and they depend on the type of outcome measure used (counting people, taking measurements on people, or time-to-event data).[4-9] For randomised phase II trials with a direct comparison between the experimental and control groups, the sample size methods are usually the same as for phase III trials.

When estimating sample size for a 'time-to-event' endpoint in a single arm trial, one approach is to use the 'counting people' category, allowing the use of simpler methods. If the median time-to-event (e.g. disease progression) is known we convert it to an event-free rate (e.g. no progression) at a specific time point, assuming an exponential distribution. Suppose the expected median time to progression using the new treatment is 8 months but the 6-month progression-free rate is required, then:

- Event-free rate at y months (P) = exponential $[(\log_e 0.5 \times y)/\text{median time}]$
- Event-free rate at six months = exponential $[(\log_e 0.5 \times 6)/8] = 0.59$ or 59%
  (the progression (event) rate at six months = $100 - 59\% = 41\%$).

If the expected median using standard therapy is 5 months, the 6-month progression-free rate is 44%. The sample size for a single-arm trial can be estimated using 59% (target) versus 44% (lowest acceptable response), which is about 70 patients.[9]

If an event rate is available but investigators wish to compare two medians, each median can be estimated by $[(\log_e 0.5)/(\log_e P)] \times y$ months.

4.5 Stopping early for toxicity

A **stopping guideline** for toxicity could be incorporated. The trial might need to stop early if the number of participants who suffer from serious treatment-related adverse events is too high. The investigators and/or the Independent Data Monitoring Committee (page 187) should examine adverse events during their regular reviews,[#] which may occur every 6 or 12 months. There are various ways to implement a safety monitoring plan. Table 4.2 shows an example using a pre-specified unacceptable toxicity rate of >25%. After the first 15 participants are treated and followed up, if 4 experience a clinically important adverse event (27%), this could trigger more careful monitoring. The likelihood of seeing 8 or more events by chance alone among 15 participants is 0.02 *if (assuming) the underlying rate were* 25%. Because this is a small probability (less than 5%), it can be concluded that the true toxicity rate is likely to exceed 25%. Consideration could then be given to stopping early. If we had seen 6 events among 15 people, although this is 40%

Table 4.2 Example of a safety monitoring plan after every 5 participants are recruited, where a toxicity rate larger than 25% is considered unacceptable.

Number of people treated	Number of important adverse events to trigger a more careful ongoing review	Number of events needed to consider stopping the trial early*	P-value*
15	4	8	0.02
20	5	9	0.04
25	6	11	0.03
30	7-8	12	0.05

* Comes from a binomial distribution.

[#]Sometimes only the IDMC will do this, especially for randomised trials and those that use blinding (higher than the 25% limit), this could still occur by chance alone in this small number of participants when the underlying rate is 25% (p-value is 0.15, which is not <0.05).

Investigators and the IDMC must examine the adverse events carefully, including severity, how long they lasted, how easily the events were treated and whether people needed to be hospitalised, and whether only a few patients experienced them but multiple times. These are balanced with signs of efficacy (benefit).

4.6 Statistical analyses

A description of the enrolled participants should be provided as a table summarising baseline characteristics, such as the age and gender distribution and other factors relevant to the disease of interest (e.g. disease stage).

Efficacy and adverse events can be analysed on an **intention-to-treat** basis, i.e. trial participants are included in the analysis whether or not they actually took the new treatment (see Section 6.5 page 102). Alternatively, investigators may only analyse participants who started the trial treatment (**safety analysis dataset**) or took enough of it (**per-protocol analysis**). The choice between these two types of analysis is largely personal preference. However, a per-protocol analysis is more likely to give the experimental therapy the best chance of success, and a better idea of its direct effect on efficacy and harms, hence both types of analyses could be provided.#

In research, '**population**' refers to the set of all people of interest and to whom a new intervention could be given. There is the concept of a **true effect**, which is meant to be a single number that applies to this population. We therefore use a trial to estimate what this true effect might be, acknowledging that the trial was only conducted on a **sample** of people.

The following focuses on analyses for single-arm phase II trials. Chapter 6 covers analyses for randomised studies.

Analysing outcome measures based on counting people

The summary statistic is a simple percentage or proportion. Box 4.4 shows an example.[15] The observed response rate is 68%.

What could the true treatment effect be?

An estimate of the **true** or **population** proportion is needed. The true value is unlikely to be 68% exactly, but it is hoped that it would be close.

The standard error of the true proportion tries to quantify how far the observed value is expected to be from the true value, given the results of the trial with a certain sample size. (This is done using assumptions about the data and established mathematical properties.) A standard error is used to produce a **confidence interval**. A trial based on every relevant participant ever would yield the true proportion. There would be no uncertainty so the standard error would be zero.

We calculate a **confidence interval (CI)** for the true proportion:

95% CI = observed proportion $\pm$ 1.96# $\times$ standard error

---

For phase III trials, intention-to-treat is the standard approach
For moderate to large studies, the multiplier '1.96' is associated with using a two-sided 95% range. Different multipliers are needed for different levels of confidence, e.g. 1.645 for a 90% CI.

Box 4.4 Example of a single-arm phase II trial. Source: Lee *et al*.[15]

Population: Newly diagnosed patients with small cell lung cancer, not previously treated

Intervention: 100 mg thalidomide orally once per day, during standard chemotherapy and afterwards as single agent maintenance therapy

Control: none

Outcome measure: Tumour response rate (complete or partial remission)

Sample size: Thalidomide should have a response rate greater than 45% (standard treatments). A value as large as 70% would indicate that it would be worthwhile investigating further. A sample size of 24 patients was required to detect this difference (80% power and one-sided 5% level of statistical significance).

Results: 25 patients were recruited of whom 17 had a tumour response.
Response rate = 68% (17/25)
One-sided 95% confidence interval (CI): lower limit is 50%
Two-sided 95% CI = 46 to 85%

Interpretation: The observed response rate was high (68%). The one-sided lower limit is 50%. This means that enough patients had a tumour response (17) to suggest that thalidomide could be associated with a true rate that is greater than the lowest acceptable rate of 45%. The observed rate is also close to the target rate of 70%. The two-sided CI indicates that the true rate could be as high as 85%.

Recommendation: Thalidomide is worth further investigation.

If the response rate is 68% (17/25), the **95% CI** is 46 to 85%[#] (formulae are easily found on the web, online calculators or standard textbooks). From this particular trial, the best estimate of the <u>true</u> proportion of responders is 68%, but there is a high certainty that the true value lies somewhere between 46 and 85%. A conservative estimate is that 46% of all participants are expected to respond, but as many as 85% could respond.

95% Confidence interval

A confidence interval indicates what the **true** value might be, based on the observed data. This true value is any summary statistic: true proportion, true mean, true time-to-event rate, true median time- to- event etc. If confidence intervals were calculated from many different studies of a similar size and design, 95% of them should contain the true value (if the assumptions used to calculate the intervals were correct), and 5% would not just by chance. There is nothing special about '95%', it is commonly used by convention; sometimes 90 or 99% CIs are used.

This is a **two-sided** CI and one that is most commonly reported. However, the design of phase II studies typically uses **one-sided** statistical significance levels, so strictly speaking, the CIs should also be one-sided. For this, only the upper or lower limit is needed, depending on which direction indicates benefit in relation to standard therapy.

[#]This is an 'exact' CI.

The standard error and, therefore, the width of the CI depend on the number of trial participants and events. The larger the study, the greater the confidence that the observed estimate is closer to the true value, so the range becomes narrower. Having few participants or events produces a wide CI, reflecting uncertainty over the true value. Conclusions based on wide CIs (e.g. 95% CI 5 to 60%) are difficult to interpret because the possible true proportion could be very low or high.

Once the 95% CI is estimated, it is examined to see if it contains the response rate for standard treatment. When there are two or more new treatments, each 95% CI is examined to observe which exclude and which include the expected effect for the standard treatment.

Could the observed result be a chance finding in this one particular study?

This question addresses statistical significance and p-values (covered in more detail in Chapter 6). These are more relevant when comparing outcomes between trial arms. However, it is possible to calculate a one-sided p-value that is consistent with the design parameters.

Using the example shown in Figure 4.2, suppose we observed 13 responses out of 44 participants (which is 29.5%). A one-sided p-value is 0.057. This means that we could see an effect as big as 29.5% or larger just by chance alone, in almost 6 in every 100 trials of a similar size and design, assuming that the true (underlying) response rate is only 20% (the lowest acceptable rate). Interpreting $p = 0.057$ must be done using the statistical significance value used in the sample size estimation, which is 0.10 (10%). Here, it is less than 0.10, so the result (29.5%) is **statistically significant** – and the trial has successfully met its objective. Investigators should not make the mistake of comparing their calculated p-value with the standard value of 0.05 (5%) used for phase III trials.

Analysing outcome measures based on taking measurements on people

When the endpoint involves taking measurements on people, the data can often be summarised by the **mean** and **standard deviation** (Chapter 2).

In the same way that a single proportion observed in a trial will be an estimate of the true proportion, an observed mean value from a trial will be an estimate of the **true mean**. The **standard error** of the mean quantifies how far the observed mean is expected to be from the true value, and is used to estimate a CI for the true mean, that has the same underlying interpretation as before:

$$95\% \, CI = \text{observed mean} \pm 1.96 \times \text{standard error}$$

Standard deviation and standard error are often confused, but they have different meanings:

- Standard deviation indicates how much the **data are naturally spread** out about the mean value (i.e. natural variability between people).
- Standard error relates not to the spread of the data, but to the **precision** of the **estimate** of the true **summary statistic** (e.g. mean value, or proportion), given the sample size.

An example of a randomised arm trial that used a continuous outcome measure is given in Box 4.5.[16] The figure is useful because it shows how the endpoint changes over time.

Box 4.5 Example of a randomised phase II trial. Source: Fox et al.[16]/ figure reproduced with permission from the Massachusetts Medical Society/ NEJM

Population: Primary or secondary progressive (i.e. relapsed) multiple sclerosis

Intervention: ≤100 mg ibudilast orally once per day, for 96 weeks

Control: Placebo orally once per day, for 96 weeks

Outcome measure: Brain atrophy, quantified by the brain parenchymal fraction (brain size relative to the volume of the outer surface contour of the brain, assessed with MRI scans)

Sample size: 125 patients per arm was specified, to find a 33–36% relative reduction in brain atrophy with 80% power and one-sided 10% level of statistical significance.

Results: 255 patients were recruited. Brain atrophy measurements over time reduced at a lower rate with ibudilast than placebo, and this was statistically significant. The results corresponded to a relative reduction of 48%, which exceeds the target effect.

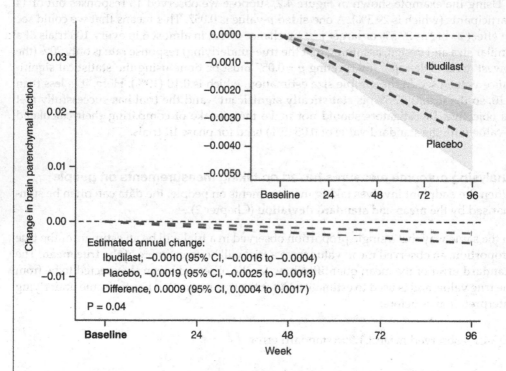

Interpretation: The observed effect seemed promising. More patients on ibudilast experienced gastrointestinal adverse effects and depression.

Recommendation: Ibudilast is worth further investigation especially using a more clinically relevant endpoint that reflects neurologic disability.

Analysing outcome measures based on time-to-event data

When the endpoint involves measuring the time until an event occurs, a Kaplan–Meier plot is derived from which a median time or event rate (proportion) at a specific time point can be obtained (see Figure 2.3, page 23), and a 95%CI can be calculated for these summary measures to reflect the true median or true event rate.

Median time is useful when there are many events, occurring continuously throughout the follow-up period, such as in studies of patients with advanced disorders. Otherwise, it can be skewed by only one or two events, and therefore be unreliable. When the median time is not reached, or it is too dependent on one or two events, the event rate at a pre-specified and clinically relevant time point might be more appropriate. Both the median and event rate come from only one point on the Kaplan-Meier curve so could be affected by chance.

Adherence and adverse events

Box 4.6 outlines how to examine adherence (compliance) and adverse events.

4.7 Interpreting phase II studies

The results of many phase II trials are used to *guide* researchers on whether a phase III trial is needed, which will eventually confirm or refute the early evidence that the new treatment might be effective. A phase II study can help to design a subsequent larger trial, in

---

Box 4.6 Reporting adherence and adverse events

Adherence

- How many participants stopped the experimental therapy early?
- Summarise the reasons why people stopped early. Does any reason stand out, e.g. toxicity, unable to swallow the size of tablet/capsule, personal or clinician choice?
- If the therapy was given continuously (e.g. daily oral drug), how long, on average, before participants stopped early?
- Did participants have the dose of the experimental therapy reduced (if so what were the reasons); and did any have dose interruptions/suspensions.
- Did taking the experimental therapy also lead to stopping of other medications normally used to treat their disease?

Adverse events

- Summarise what they were.
- What are the most common ones and how severe/serious were they?
- Are there any major uncommon events: e.g. treatment-related deaths, acute kidney/liver injury?
- Decide whether to report any severity grade of event (e.g. chronic disorders) or only more severe/high grade events (e.g. acute disorders).
- Consider providing a summary of adverse events judged to be *caused* by the new therapy.
- If there are major toxicities, how long did it take for them to occur since starting the experimental treatment?

terms of outcome measures, sample size and trial conduct. The decision to proceed to a phase III trial should be based on several efficacy endpoints, as well as adverse events, recruitment and acceptability.

Many phase II studies are conducted in a few specialist centres and by experienced health professionals. Therefore, an observed beneficial treatment effect, especially if the trial is not blind (i.e. it is open label), may not be seen in routine practice, or the effect size is over-estimated.

The findings should also be interpreted in the context of the type of participants who were enrolled. They might, for example have a lower response rate than that assumed in the sample size calculation because they had a poorer prognosis than expected; or they had a much better prognosis than anticipated hence a higher response rate was observed. Either of these could explain why a study does not meet its primary objectives. If the observed response rates are very different from those specified in the design, especially for the control arm, the investigators should attempt to find out why.

Many treatments that appear effective in phase II studies are shown to be ineffective when tested in a phase III trial. In the example in Box 4.4, a large randomised trial was conducted afterwards which showed no effect.[15, 17]

4.8 Summary points

- Phase II studies are a useful way of obtaining preliminary information about a new intervention in a relatively small number of participants.
- There are several different designs, including those that have a comparison arm.
- Participants should be monitored closely, especially for adverse effects.
- The results of phase II studies are generally descriptive, focusing on the size of the effect of the new intervention and the 95% confidence interval.
- The characteristics of participants entered into the trial should be described in sufficient detail.
- The decision to conduct a larger, confirmatory trial should depend on several factors: efficacy, safety and feasibility.
- Translational research and biomarker driven trials can be used to evaluate several novel therapies efficiently, or to evaluate a particular therapy across a range of disorder subtypes within a single trial protocol.

References

1. Scher HI, Heller G. Picking the winners in a sea of plenty. *Clin Cancer Res* 2002; **8**:400–404.
2. Lee JJ, Feng L. Randomized phase II designs in cancer clinical trials: current status and future directions. *J Clin Oncol* 2005; **23**:4450–4457.
3. Rubinstein LV, Korn EL, Friedlin B *et al*. Design issues of randomised phase II trials and a proposal for phase II screening trials. *J Clin Oncol* 2005; **23**:7199–7206.
4. A'Hern R. Sample size tables for exact single-stage phase II designs. *Stat Med* 2001; **20**:859–866.
5. Machin D, Campbell M, Tan SB, Tan SH. *Sample Size Tables for Clinical Studies*. 3rd edn, Wiley-Blackwell Science, 2009 [comes with free software].
6. PS: Power and Sample size Calculation. https://ps-power-and-sample-size-calculation. software.informer.com/3.1/
7. Southwest Oncology Group (SWOG). https://stattools.crab.org/

8. PASS (Power Analysis and Sample Size software). `http://www.ncss.com`
9. nQuery. `http://www.statsols.com`
10. Cannistra SA. Phase II trials in Journal of Clinical Oncology. J Clin Oncol 2009; **27**(19):3073–3076.
11. Ledermann JA, Hackshaw A, Kaye S *et al*. A randomized phase II placebo-controlled trial of maintenance therapy using the oral triple angiokinase inhibitor BIBF 1120 following chemotherapy for relapsed ovarian cancer. JCO 2011; **29**:3798–3804.
12. Park JJH, Hsu G, Siden EG, Thorlund K, Mills EJ. An overview of precision oncology basket and umbrella trials for clinicians. CA Cancer J Clin 2020; **70**(2):125–137.
13. Hyman DM, Puzanov I, Subbiah V *et al*. Vemurafenib in multiple nonmelanoma cancers with BRAF V600 mutations. N Engl J Med 2015; **373**(8):726–736.
14. Turner NC, Kingston B, Kilburn LS *et al*. Circulating tumour DNA analysis to direct therapy in advanced breast cancer (plasmaMATCH): a multicentre, multicohort, phase 2a, platform trial. Lancet Oncol 2020; **21**(10):1296–1308.
15. Lee S-M, Buchler T, James L *et al*. Phase II trial of carboplatin and etoposide with thalidomide in patients with poor prognosis small-cell lung cancer. *Lung Cancer* 2008; **59**(3):364–368.
16. Fox RJ, Coffey CS, Conwit R *et al*. NN102/SPRINT-MS trial investigators. Phase 2 trial of Ibudilast in progressive multiple sclerosis. N Engl J Med 2018; **379**(9):846–855.
17. Lee SM, Woll PJ, Rudd R *et al*. Anti-angiogenic therapy using thalidomide combined with chemotherapy in small cell lung cancer: a randomized, double-blind, placebo-controlled trial. J Natl Cancer Inst 2009; **101**(15):1049–1057.

CHAPTER 5

Phase III trials: design

A randomised controlled phase III trial should provide enough evidence to warrant a change in practice. Key design features were outlined in Chapter 1 which are covered in more detail here. This chapter provides an overview of the main types of objectives, common designs, specific considerations of the main design components (population, intervention, control and outcome: PICO), non-inferiority and multiplicity. In addition to specific references for this chapter, several more are given on page 205 (further reading).

5.1 Trial objectives

The main objective of a phase III study is usually based on **efficacy**, **safety** or both. Occasionally, it might be health-related quality of life when it is considered as an efficacy measure. Other trials aim to improve how healthcare is delivered, so the endpoints used might reflect some performance measure (e.g. shorter waiting times in a clinic). Box 5.1 shows the three fundamental trial objectives.

There are also **bioequivalence trials**, in which two forms of the same drug, for example, produced using a new method or a different formulation, are compared. All that may be required is to determine that a similar amount of drug is taken into the body (i.e. similar bioavailability), and this can be done using a biochemical marker or other surrogate.

5.2 Designs

Common trial designs are illustrated in Figure 5.1, and the fundamental aspects are in Figure 1.3 (page 8). National regulators provide guidance on trial design, with a focus on investigational drugs.[1, 2]

Most trials have **parallel groups**: each group of participants receives only one intervention. For chronic disorders, where the desired outcome is a relief of symptoms rather than a disease cure, it is possible to allocate both the new and standard treatment to the same participant in sequence (**crossover trial**) or at the same time (**split-person**). Instead of randomly allocating participants to treatment arms, the ordering of treatments is random so that a similar number of people given treatment A first are given treatment B first. The strength of a crossover study is that each participant acts as his/her own control comparison, and the sample size is smaller than required for a parallel group trial.[3]

Crossover designs have limitations. There should be no **residual (carryover) effect** from the first treatment that influences the response to the second treatment because this could make it difficult to compare their effects reliably. To minimise this problem, a sufficiently long **washout period** is required – a time between the two trial treatments

A Concise Guide to Clinical Trials, Second Edition. Allan Hackshaw.
© 2024 John Wiley & Sons Ltd. Published 2024 by John Wiley & Sons Ltd.

Box 5.1 Trial objectives

Comparing two interventions, A and B
(B could be the standard treatment, placebo or no intervention)

Superiority	A is more effective (beneficial) than B
Equivalence	A has a similar effect to B
Non-inferiority	A is not much less effective than B (and it could have a similar effect or be better)

'Effect' is associated with any primary trial endpoint, such as death, occurrence or recurrence of a disorder or measure of symptoms.

Equivalence and non-inferiority trials are conducted when the new intervention is expected to have fewer side effects, be more cost-effective, have improved quality of life or be more convenient to administer or appealing.

---

when neither is given. The washout period duration depends on the aetiology of the disorder and the pharmacological properties of the trial treatments. There may also be a **period effect**, in that the ordering of the treatments matters: people who have A then B respond differently to those who have B then A. This can be allowed for in the statistical analysis. If there is uncertainty over the strength of the carryover or period effects, a standard two-arm trial is preferred.

Pragmatic trials are meant to have minimal (broad) eligibility criteria to reflect the target population more closely, interventions that are easier to administer (and not usually blinded), and assessments of participants that are standard routine practice (i.e. no/few extra clinic visits or additional tests or scans). Only essential follow-up and outcome data are often collected, e.g. mainly from electronic health records.

Figure 5.1 also shows examples of multi-arm trials. A special case is a **factorial trial** which involves two new interventions, each compared with a control arm. This is an efficient design because it avoids having two separate two-arm trials. There are two distinct contexts: one in which the treatments should not interact with each other, and the other in which an interaction is expected. An interaction occurs if the combined effect of A and B differs from what would be expected by adding the effects seen when A and B are given separately (see page 116). The trial would have to be larger to incorporate an interaction effect than if no interaction were assumed. Figure 5.1 shows an example of a trial that evaluated folic acid and a multivitamin combination for preventing neural tube defects among pregnant women.[4] The following comparisons could be made:

- B + D versus A + C (Is folic acid effective?)
- C + D versus A + B (Are multivitamins effective?)
- D versus B (Is folic acid plus multivitamins better than folic acid alone?)
- D versus C (Is folic acid plus multivitamins better than multivitamins alone?)
- Plus comparisons with the control only (A).

Adaptive designs

Adaptive designs can help make clinical trials more efficient, especially when they allow the evaluation of multiple interventions for a disorder.[5–7] They involve altering parts of the design during the study in a formalised way. A **platform trial** of multiple treatments

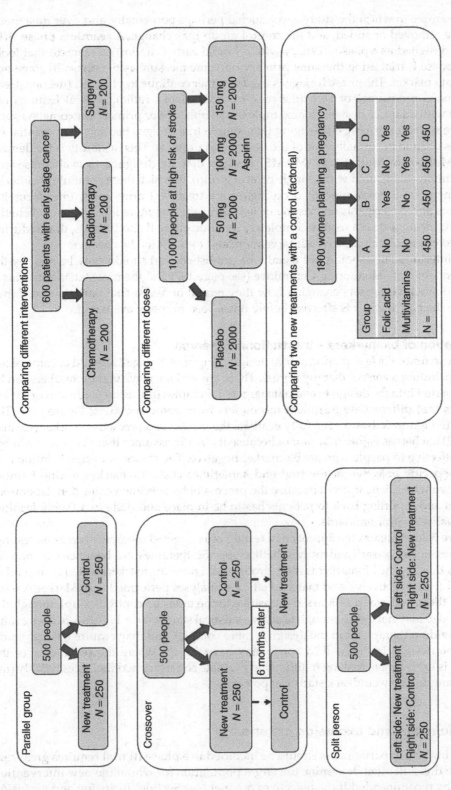

Figure 5.1 Illustration of phase III trial designs. Left side: two-arm unpaired (parallel) or paired data (crossover or split-person) studies. Right side: multi-arm trials. Solid arrows indicate the randomisation.

is an example in which the study is conducted perhaps perpetually, and over time therapies are removed or added, and the control group may change. A **seamless phase II/III trial** is designed as a phase III study with a formal early (interim) assessment that looks like a phase II trial using the same primary outcome measure as the phase III stage or a surrogate marker. The phase II stage is used to either continue to phase III (the new treatment looks promising) or stop (the new treatment looks futile). Several features can change with adaptive designs, for example the sample size or primary outcome. As such, they are statistically more challenging than simple trial designs because the potential for changes need to be formally part of the design and protocol. This flexibility is fundamental to **Multi-Arm Multi-Stage (MAMS) designs** that are designed to evaluate several interventions (compared with a single control group), in which there are multiple interim assessments of efficacy used to drop ineffective treatment arms early, thus focussing resources and participants on existing or new arms that are more likely to show benefit.[8] Adaptive designs do not require completely separate phase II and III trials, thus reducing the time taken to evaluate a new intervention, and they should be cheaper.

The interim results should not usually be published, and should only be seen by the Independent Data Monitoring Committee (see page 187) and the trial statistician. This is to avoid site investigators changing how they recruit or assess trial participants, if they assume the new therapy is effective before it has been properly evaluated.

Integration of biomarkers – translational research

Multi-arm umbrella (e.g. platform) trial designs[9] (Figure 4.5, page 47) could become phase III by including a control therapy arm(s). There are various ways that biomarkers can be incorporated into the design to evaluate targeted therapies (precision medicine) or to find markers that differentiate treatment responders from non-responders; Figure 5.2.[10] The design in Figures 5.2b and c can fully evaluate the marker as a predictive marker (see also page 121), whereas Figure 5.2a cannot because it already assumes that the new treatment is not effective in people who are biomarker negative. The choice of design is influenced by the specific objective of the trial and sometimes costs. Biomarker testing is more expensive when done upfront because the process of biospecimen collection, laboratory analysis and reporting back to patients has to be in place and done in a timely fashion, with quality control standards.

Figure 5.2d evaluates the approach of testing plus targeted therapies versus no testing, and does not necessarily identify whether specific therapies are beneficial or not. To address this, the 'no biomarker testing' group could have the markers tested at the end of the trial (retrospectively), and matched efficacy analyses performed (e.g. Marker A positives in the tested group vs Marker A positive in the untested control group), though the sample size may not be big enough to show statistical significance. Figure 5.2e does evaluate individual therapies, but the design is more complex and may require a larger study size. The designs in Figure 5.2d and e may have groups where the prevalence of the marker is uncommon, making it difficult to evaluate some targeted therapies reliably (the small sample size would lack statistical power).

5.3 Inclusion and exclusion criteria

Specifying which participants should be included in a phase III trial requires great care because this will often determine the target population for whom the new intervention would be recommended if the objectives are met (see Section 'Inclusion and exclusion

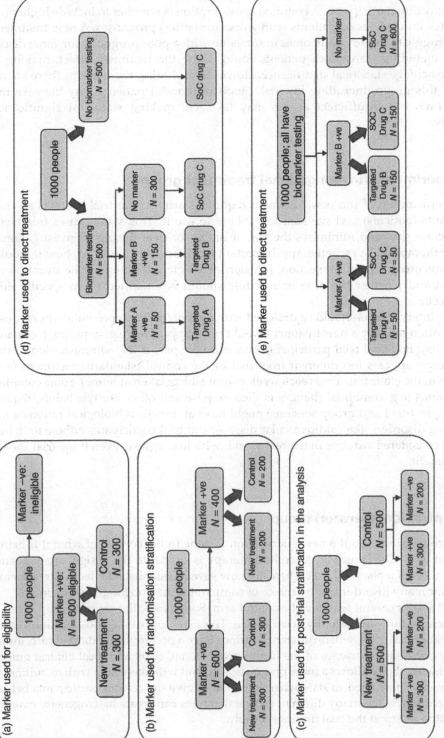

Figure 5.2 Trial designs that incorporate a biomarker that is integral to the interpretation of the treatment effect. SoC: standard of care. +ve: positive (e.g. genetic mutation), –ve: negative. Solid arrows indicate the randomisation. The marker testing is done upfront (prospectively) and in real time in all designs except 5c, where the laboratory analyses can be done retrospectively at the end of the study on stored biospecimens. In 5e, people who have no marker in their biospecimens (or imaging scans) could either all have SoC or they could be randomised between SoC and another investigational therapy.

criteria', page 7). Only essential eligibility criteria should be specified, and other selection criteria could be listed as desirable or phrased in a way to allow some flexibility when recruiting participants. A common consideration is whether to include higher (or lower) risk individuals or patients with worse (or better) prognoses. A new treatment might struggle to improve outcomes in someone with a poor prognosis for some disorders, so including many such patients could dilute the treatment effect, making it harder to achieve statistical significance. However, excluding them means there are no data for this group. Including low-risk (good prognosis) patients may increase the accrual rate, but insufficient events may be seen, making statistical significance less likely.

5.4 Experimental/investigational treatment group

The administration of the new treatment requires clarity in the trial protocol so that participants (patients) and site staff know how to use it. This standardises treatment policy across sites and minimises the risk of under- or over-dosing of investigational drugs or therapies like radiotherapy. Important items are: when to start, how it would be administered (e.g. oral, injection, infusion or surgical technique), the duration of treatment and whether the dose or schedule should be modified when specific side effects occur.

Ideally, interventions should be designed with patient/public representatives because they can often see why a new treatment would be unappealing (e.g. requiring too many clinic visits). Potential trial participants may not take part if the administration of the new therapy appears too different from that of the control (standard) treatment (e.g. infusions in the clinic four times each week vs oral tablets taken at home). Some complex interventions (e.g. combined changes in diet, exercise and other lifestyle habits, requiring multiple 1-to-1 and group sessions) might have an excellent biological rationale for preventing disorders like cardiovascular disease, and trial participants adhere to it, but could be considered arduous in the real-world, with low uptake, even if the trial shows a clear benefit.

5.5 Control (comparator) group

Making conclusions about a new intervention is done in the context of what it is being compared with. The choice of the control therapy is crucial to the design, analysis and interpretation of a phase III trial. There are now several established effective treatments options for many disorders so the choice of comparator may no longer be obvious.

Box 5.2 shows several features of a control arm. Sometimes, the control group is not a single therapy, but **clinician/physician choice**. This can be advantageous for multicentre and multinational trials, where different locations have a preferred standard of care, influenced by personal experience of the health professional, costs and local clinical guidelines. Clinician choice allows a more pragmatic trial and will likely help with recruitment. However, sites may need to state what they plan to give the control participants before recruitment starts. Too many different control therapies can create heterogeneity making it difficult to interpret the trial findings reliably.

Box 5.2 Choosing the control (comparator) intervention

What makes a good comparator?

* Placebo alone, when there are no current standards of care, and endpoints are subjective
* Placebo plus standard of care so that participants are not deprived of anything
* The comparator is a current standard of care that participants would have
* Participants will accept the control therapy if they are randomised to it
* Health professionals are willing to randomise participants to the control therapy

What makes an *inappropriate* comparator (new therapy might appear more effective than it really is)?

* Control therapy is rarely or no longer used in current practice in many locations, and it may be known to have less efficacy than other treatments
* Control therapy dose is too low
* Control therapy dose is too high, leading to more side effects and early stopping, so patients do not get the expected benefit
* Substandard treatment: placebo instead of an active drug
* Inferior (substandard) delivery of the control therapy: e.g. tablets instead of an injection of the same drug formulation might have less efficacy

---

5.6 Randomisation and allocating participants (see page 10)

Most trials have a similar number of participants in each arm (**equal** or **1:1 randomisation**). Sometimes, more participants are required in one arm (**unequal randomisation**), usually the new intervention, such as a ratio of 2:1. This may be because more reliable data are needed on adverse events. Also, participants may be more likely to participate in a trial if they perceive a 2 in 3 chance of getting a potentially more effective treatment, rather than a 50% chance with 1:1 allocation.

For the same sample size, statistical power associated with comparing two trial arms decreases as the allocation ratio becomes more unequal. To prevent loss of power, unequal randomisation is therefore specified in the sample size calculation, resulting in a larger study size.

Allocating individuals or groups of individuals to the trial groups

Randomising individual participants into different groups is the preferred approach. However, *groups* of participants may be randomly allocated instead. An example would be a trial to determine whether a new educational programme for teenagers could reduce their prevalence of smoking and alcohol drinking. The programme would be compared with no intervention (control). If teenagers were randomised within the same school (or class) to either the programme or control, they would mix with each other and share their experiences of the programme. The effect of the programme could then be diluted. Also, the teenagers would have to be separated to deliver the programme to some and not others, which may have practical difficulties.

An alternative is to randomise schools. All teenagers in one school receive the new programme, and all those in another school become the control group. Several schools

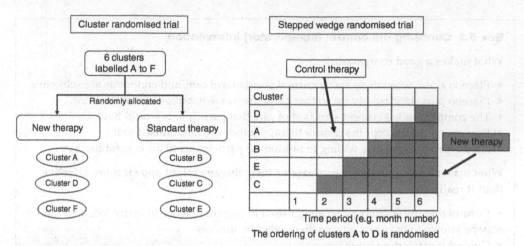

Figure 5.3 Standard cluster and stepped wedge cluster randomised trials (a cluster is any defined group of people, e.g. hospital, school or primary care clinic). In the stepped wedge design, participants in Cluster C receive the control intervention for only one time period and then the new intervention for five time periods; in contrast to Cluster D who have the control therapy for five time periods then the new intervention for only one period. The stepped wedge approach allows the new intervention to be rolled out gradually across sites making it more feasible.

would need to be randomised in this way, and it is often a more practical way of delivering both interventions. This is called a **cluster randomised trial**,[11] and a special case is a **stepped wedge design**[12] (Figure 5.3). They are particularly suited for interventions that cannot be blinded. Data are still obtained from each trial participant, but both the sample size calculation and statistical analysis allow for the clustering, i.e. that participants *within* a cluster are more likely to be correlated with each other in terms of characteristics and how they respond to the intervention (intraclass correlation), than participants *between* clusters. This makes the sample size larger than when randomising individuals.

5.7 Blinding (placebo)

Using a placebo is often considered to be a gold standard, particularly when some of the trial endpoints have a subjective element. Where ethical and feasible, placebo (including sham devices and surgical procedures) is preferred. Many decision-makers evaluate the potential for bias in confirmatory practice-changing trials, and placebo-controlled studies tend to have minimal bias. Placebos should not be able to induce a response.

5.8 Outcome measures

The main outcome measure(s) needs to persuade health professionals to change practice (see also section 2.1 on page 15). It will often be obvious, for example death, the occurrence or recurrence of a specific disease, or endpoints for disease/symptom control used and accepted many times previously. Otherwise, validated endpoints should be used as long as they are specific to the disorder of interest (e.g. the Beck Depression Inventory [BDI] or the Montgomery–Asberg Depression Rating Scale [MADRS] for measuring symptoms of depression).

Examples of **objective measures** are death or well-defined disorders that are clinically diagnosed using standard methods such as scans or biopsies (e.g. having a stroke or cancer), or standard physiological or biochemical measurements (e.g. blood pressure or lipid levels). **Subjective measures** are those reported by the participant, such as symptoms or health-related quality of life, or visual/physical assessments made by a health professional.

Below are four possible endpoints in a randomised trial of a flu vaccine in the elderly to illustrate how to consider the strengths and limitations of endpoints:[13]

1. Serological evidence of the flu virus, i.e. an increase in antibodies against influenza detected in a blood sample 5 months after the vaccination (measured in a laboratory).
2. Diagnosis by a family doctor after the person presented with flu-like symptoms
3. Self-reported flu-like symptoms using a questionnaire completed by the participants
4. Hospital admission for respiratory disease (not used in the trial[13]).

'Serological evidence' is an **objective measure** that should be unaffected by a lack of blinding and measured reliably, so it might be the most preferred. However, some individuals with antibodies may feel perfectly well, and others are not unwell enough to visit their doctor, so the clinical relevance of this endpoint is uncertain.

'Diagnosis by clinician' is part subjective and objective. The clinician uses standardised criteria to help classify people as having flu or not, but this still requires some judgement. It might be considered clinically relevant because these people have felt so unwell that they decided to visit their doctor. They are more likely to go to hospital for respiratory problems or die from flu. Knowing whether the person had the vaccine or not could affect (bias) the clinical diagnosis of flu, hence the value of using placebo.

'Self-reported flu' requires participants to complete a questionnaire at home, and then a central reviewer classifies them as having flu or not according to a set of criteria. However, it is a **subjective measure** that may have wide variability which could mask or dilute the treatment effect. If participants are not blind to treatment, those given the vaccine may be less likely to report flu-related symptoms thinking they do not have flu. Those not given the vaccine may be more likely to report these symptoms, which may be unrelated to the flu, because they perceive they have had no protection. This bias would make the vaccine seem effective when it is not, or to over-estimate the effect. Self-reported flu might appear to be the weakest endpoint, but it could reflect a societal impact because individuals who think they have flu (whether they actually have it or not) are likely to take time off work and buy (expensive) over-the-counter medications.

'Hospital admission for respiratory disease' would be associated with the most severely affected patients. It might be less affected by a lack of blinding. It relies on being notified of all admissions of the trial participants. The clinical relevance is clear because it is linked to flu-related morbidity and mortality. However, the proportion of elderly people admitted to hospital for or who die from flu-related respiratory disorders is relatively low, so a large trial is needed to see sufficient events for a reliable evaluation.

Dealing with subjective measures

For outcomes that involve some degree of subjectivity (e.g., evaluating brain scans for evidence of dementia progression or non-progression), it is worthwhile considering the value, feasibility and costs of having either (i) two local independent assessors or (ii) a **blinded independent central review** (BICR) where a central assessor(s) who is unaware of the local assessment examines the primary outcome for all trial participants, a random sample of all participants or all those who had the event of interest plus a random sample of those who did not. Such procedures could strengthen the reliability of the endpoint assessment and ultimately the treatment effect, but they can be expensive.

Composite outcome measures

Some endpoints consist of several event types (components) combined into one, called a **composite endpoint**.[14,15] An example comes from trials of primary or secondary cardiovascular disease prevention which often use an endpoint with three components: fatal cardiovascular death, non-fatal myocardial infarction or non-fatal stroke (called 3P-MACE: Major Adverse Cardiac Event). Composite endpoints avoid having to deal with several separate outcome measures, and they increase the number of events, making it easier to achieve statistical significance either for detecting a treatment benefit or to show non-inferiority. It is assumed that the investigational therapy has a beneficial effect on all components, but this is often not the case in reality.

The component events usually have equal 'weight', for example it is assumed that a non-fatal myocardial infarction is as important as death from stroke. Also, only the first occurrence of any of the events is used for each participant, because the clinical management may influence the risk of any subsequent event that occurred afterwards. An alternative approach is the **win ratio** that considers multiple events per participant in the analysis after the investigators rank the clinical importance of each component event.[16]

A composite endpoint is defined upfront in the protocol. Sometimes components are added during the trial because the event rate is lower than expected using the initial definition. An example is changing the endpoint from 3P-MACE to 4P-MACE that includes hospitalisation for unstable angina. Although expanding the composite outcome leads to more events, it could dilute the treatment difference if the new therapy has little/no effect on the added item(s), and statistical significance becomes more difficult to achieve. Components can also be removed, perhaps to strengthen the endpoint as long as the number of expected events is not compromised. Modifying a composite endpoint should not be done after looking at interim efficacy results.

Clarifying outcome measures – estimands

An **Estimand** (what is to be estimated) aims to provide greater clarity of outcome measures by combining key attributes of design and analysis.[17, 18] It can consist of four components (Box 5.3), and different statistical analyses (strategies) would be represented as additional columns.

5.9 Participant follow-up

Box 1.5 (page 11) summarises how data in trials can be collected. The follow-up length must be enough for the new intervention to produce a beneficial response. For 'counting people' or time-to-event outcomes, we also require a sufficient number of events to ensure statistical significance.

For trials of chronic disorders and behavioural change interventions, follow-up should be long enough to see whether benefits can be maintained or not. An expensive new

Box 5.3 Two examples of simple estimands

	Example 1[19]	Example 2[20]
Component:	Secukinumab (new) versus fumaric acid ester (control)	Crizotinib (new) versus standard chemotherapy (control)
Population (main eligibility criteria)	Adults with plaque psoriasis	Advanced non-small cell lung cancer, with ALK-positive tumours
Variable (quantitative endpoint)	Change from baseline to 24 weeks in the Dermatology Life Quality Index (DLQI).	Overall survival (time to death from any cause)
Intercurrent event*	Change treatment to alternative non-trial therapy before 24 weeks, if either trial treatment fails. Not accounted for in the analysis.	Patients on chemotherapy are allowed to switch to crizotinib if their tumour progresses. These patients will be censored at the time of switching.
Summary measure (effect size)	Mean difference: mean change in DLQI from baseline using secukinumab minus mean change from baseline using fumaric acid from linear regression.	Overall survival compared between the two groups using hazard ratio from Cox regression.

*Dealing with events that affect the interpretation of the treatment effect (e.g. salvage therapies given if the disease worsens, subsequent lines of therapies, non-adherence to the trial treatments or switching interventions).

therapy for plaque psoriasis might lead to an improvement in skin condition for the first 4 weeks, but if the effect wears off with little/no benefit over standard therapy beyond 24 weeks, this might make it less appealing.

How participants are assessed during follow-up needs to be the same for all trial arms but sometimes this is not possible (e.g. the new and control treatments are delivered at different times). If one trial group are assessed more frequently than another, this could bias outcomes (e.g. more reporting of adverse events) simply because they are asked more often about their health. Telephone assessments can minimise this issue.

The frequency and type of follow-up assessments will affect the trial costs and feasibility at sites, especially if many visits are in addition to routine practice or some assessments are expensive, time consuming or non-standard.

5.10 Estimating study size

Several elements determine sample size (Figure 5.4):

Effect size: the estimated (expected) effect of the new treatment.

Statistical significance (error rate, or type I error or α-level): the likelihood of observing a treatment effect and concluding superiority (or non-inferiority) but the new treatment is truly not superior (or truly not non-inferior) - the conclusion is wrong.

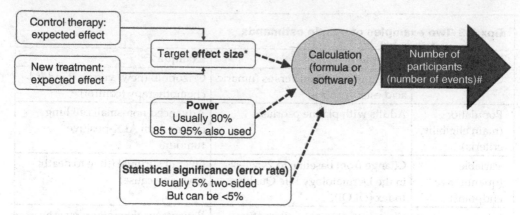

Figure 5.4 Information needed to calculate the sample size. *e.g. relative risk, odds ratio, absolute risk difference, hazard ratio, mean difference. # For time-to-event (event driven) endpoints. The sample size method depends on the type of outcome measure (counting people, taking measurements on people or time-to-event); objective (e.g. superiority or non-inferiority) and parallel group or crossover design.

Table 5.1 Examples of sample sizes when the outcome measure is based on 'counting people' (e.g. binary outcome). The table shows how the number of participants required for a two-arm trial changes with the effect size and power (the first 4 rows use 5% two-sided statistical significance, the bottom row uses 1%).

Response rate (%)		Effect size	Power (%)		
Control therapy	New therapy	Risk difference (percentage points)	80	85	90
50	60	10	776	886	1038
50	70	20	186	214	248
50	80	30	78	88	104
50	90	40	40	44	52
50	90	40	60	66	74

Power (1 minus type II error or β-level): the likelihood of finding the target effect size (or greater) in the trial *and* that the result is statistically significant, when the treatment truly is superior (or truly non-inferior) - the conclusion is correct.

Table 5.1 shows example of sample sizes. Large treatment effects require small trials, and small treatment effects require large trials. Trial size increases for:

- smaller effect sizes
- higher power
- smaller statistical significance.

The sample size estimate only reflects the contributing assumptions. If the assumptions are unrealistic, the trial size will be too small or too large. Because the target effect size is influenced by the control therapy effect, the choice of the comparator is crucial and should not be done to deliberately make the effect size large (see Box 5.2).

Expected effect size

The term **effect size** is used to compare an endpoint between two trial groups (Box 5.4). It could be a relative risk, risk difference, hazard ratio or difference between two means (Sections 6.1–6.4 on pages 79 to 88).

Box 5.4 Considerations about effect sizes when estimating trial size

- Sample size is greatly influenced by the expected effect size.
- Sample size methods use estimates (guesses) of the effect size which investigators often over-estimate.
- Effect size should be any of the following:
  - realistic and achievable, e.g. estimated from prior evidence/studies
  - clinically useful
  - the minimum clinically important effect
- Choose a realistic effect size first then look at sample size.
- *Do not choose a sample size first, then say what the corresponding effect size is (the trial could be underpowered for a smaller effect).*
- Consider time and cost to recruit and follow-up participants.
- Primary statistical analysis should be based on the same method used in the sample size calculation.

When the outcome measure is based on counting people, the expected percentage (or risk) is specified for each trial arm. The sample size depends on the actual value of the percentages. For example, the sample size comparing 10 versus 15% is 1372 participants, but for 50 versus 55% it is 3130, even though the difference is 5 percentage points in both cases. This is because the *proportional* increase from 10 to 15% (50% increase, 15/10) is much larger than that from 50 to 55% (10% increase, 55/50), requiring a smaller study. When taking measurements on people we can use the **standardised difference** (sometimes called Cohen's *d*).

$$\text{Standardised difference} = \frac{\text{mean value in Group 1} - \text{mean in Group 2}}{\text{standard deviation of the measurement}}$$

The effect size is defined in terms of the number of standard deviation units. Therefore, if the individual means and standard deviation are unknown, investigators can directly state whether they expect a small, moderate or large standardised difference, corresponding to roughly <0.2, around 0.4 or above 0.7, respectively.

For time-to-event data, there are various methods to estimate sample size depending on how the effect size is specified (e.g. a hazard ratio, two medians or two event rates at a specific time point), and information on the length of recruitment and follow-up.

There are several sample-size methods and software.[21-25] Table 5.1 shows the dramatic reduction in study size as the effect size changes from small to large (10 to 40 percentage point risk difference). Overestimating the effect size is likely to lead to an **underpowered** study if the actual treatment effect is materially smaller (i.e. the observed result is not statistically significant, so no firm conclusions can be made).

There are also **simulation methods** which, instead of using a single formula, involve the creation of hundreds or thousands of datasets of hypothetical individuals using number generators, assuming varying study sizes and input parameters (e.g. estimates of effect in each trial arm). We then count how many datasets achieve statistical significance for certain effect sizes, to provide power and a minimum target sample size.

Allowing for participant drop-outs and missing data

When participants withdraw or are lost to follow-up some endpoints cannot be assessed for them. To allow for this, if the sample size were 500 participants and 20% were expected to withdraw, the trial would aim to recruit 625 patients [500/(1−0.20)], because 625 less 20% is 500.

Missing data can be a major problem for the final analyses, and although there are several ways of dealing with it, none are ideal and different methods can yield different results. The best approach is to minimise missing data during the trial:

- Ensure that endpoints are easy to measure by researchers, or easily extracted from medical records
- Minimise the number of variables on case report forms.

Multiple analyses of the primary outcome measure

The study design and sample size can allow for multiple formal interim analyses, but a key goal is to keep the overall error rate at <5% (statistical significance level).[14] One approach is a **group sequential design**[26] that incorporates a pre-specified number of interim analyses. At each analysis, the trial can stop early with fewer participants if the observed effect size crosses a pre-defined boundary for either superiority (the new treatment is shown to be more effective than the comparator) or a boundary indicating that the new treatment is less effective or futile. Group sequential designs tend to require more participants than those without multiple formal interim analyses.

Adaptive designs also use statistical methodology to change the study size or stop early based on formal interim analyses.[5, 6] For example:

- Start off with a small expected effect size and a large target study size, but stop the trial early with fewer participants if a larger treatment effect is found during interim analyses.
- Start off with a large expected effect size and a small target study size, then increase the number of participants if the interim analyses indicate a smaller treatment effect.

5.11 Non-inferiority and equivalence

To show that one treatment is more effective than another (superiority) is relatively straightforward. An effect size just needs to be statistically significant, and clinically meaningful. A different approach is needed to show either that two interventions have a similar effect (equivalence)[27] or non-inferiority,[28, 29] the latter is more common.

There are several reasons, other than efficacy, why a new intervention would be more appealing than a current standard: fewer side effects, cheaper, better quality of life or easier to administer. There is interest in comparing drugs in the same class (**head-to-head trials**), finding less invasive surgical techniques, or reducing the number of drugs or doses in a regimen, or reducing treatment duration.

For equivalence trials, the efficacy of a new intervention needs to be within a pre-specified range *around* the effect of a comparator. For example, if the response rate using standard of care is 60%, a new therapy could be considered equivalent if its response rate is 60% ± 5%. The '5%' is called the **equivalence limit**, and 55-65% could be called the **equivalence range**.

Non-inferiority trials require careful consideration. Assume that the true survival rate with standard therapy is 40%. A new therapy is safer. It is unlikely that the true survival rate with the new therapy is exactly 40%. A true rate higher than 40% would be ideal. However, we take a conservative approach and assume that participants (patients) would be willing to lose some efficacy for the benefits (e.g. fewer adverse events). This is essentially a trade-off. Would 39% be considered acceptable, 38 or 35%? Essentially, we ask '*How low are you willing to go?*'' before saying that the loss in efficacy is unacceptable, because it outweighs the benefits. It could be 35%, a difference of 5 percentage points. If the (true) survival rate using the new treatment is 36%, we conclude that it could be used in practice, but if it was 34% we would probably not recommend it.

This 'allowable' difference needs to be pre-specified. It is used in the sample size calculation and is essential for interpreting the trial results (see Section 7.1, page 107). It is called the **non-inferiority margin** or **maximum allowable difference**. There is no fixed rule for determining the margin, but a regulatory agency or payer may prespecify it for drug trials of particular disorders. It could be a third or half of what is considered a clinically important effect for a therapy with superior efficacy. For example, if a hazard ratio for overall survival of 0.80 represents a beneficial therapy, a non-inferiority margin could correspond to half of this gain: margin is hazard ratio of 1.11, calculated as $1/[0.8+(1-0.8)/2]$. The margin needs to preserve a minimum clinically acceptable effect of a treatment had it been compared with a placebo. But it should not be larger than an effect that would be used to determine superiority.

The non-inferiority margin requires careful consideration beyond simple numerical specification (Box 5.5). Examples are in Figure 5.5.

Sample sizes for non-inferiority and equivalence studies are larger than superiority trials because the effect size associated with the margin should be smaller than what is considered to be a clinically important effect for a superiority trial.

The study size might also be powered for expected benefits measured by secondary endpoints (e.g. a lower number of adverse events).

Box 5.5 Considerations when determining a non-inferiority margin

• What is the disorder, and how serious is it?
• How big is the numerical loss of efficacy?
• What is the consequence if someone 'fails' on the new treatment? How serious is this and what can be done for them? Is there 'salvage' therapy, is it effective, does it have serious side effects or is it expensive?
• If there is no salvage intervention for those who fail (e.g. death, or miscarriage as in Figure 5.5), the margin should be small.
• How many participants are expected to fail? If there are few failures, then having the majority of participants taking a safer/cheaper/easier to administer therapy might outweigh the few who need salvage therapy that may be harmful/expensive.
• The above are balanced against the expected benefits of the new treatment.

➢ Specifying big margins require small trials (but the margin might not be accepted generally).
➢ Specifying small margins require big trials (long and expensive).
➢ The margin must be agreed by the investigators and ideally patient/public representatives. Surveys of patients and clinicians could be used to obtain a range of acceptable margins.
➢ Ultimately, the margin must be accepted by both patients/public and health professionals who would use the new treatment in routine practice.

Rheumatoid arthritis
Standard: adalimumab (injection every 2 weeks)
New: tofacitinib (oral tablets daily).

Endpoint: 6-month response rate is 35% (American College of Rheumatology criteria) using the standard.

Non-inferiority margin 13 percentage points (i.e. the true response rate for tofacitinib can go down to 22%).

Might appear to be a large difference but patients failing to respond can be readily treated with other therapies.

HIV
Standard: antiretroviral therapy (oral tablets daily)
New: long-acting cabotegravir and rilpivirine (monthly intramuscular injections).

Endpoint: 48-week response rate is 98% (HIV-1 RNA level <50 copies/mL) using the standard.

Non-inferiority margin is 6 percentage points (i.e. the true response rate for long-acting therapy can go down to 92%).

Although non-responders can be given other treatments, the allowable margin has to be quite low because of the severity/importance of HIV resistance.

in vitro fertilisation (infertility):
administering progesterone
Standard: crinone (vaginal gel preparation, that is uncomfortable and has side effects)
New: prolutex (subcutaneous injection).

Endpoint: 10 week ongoing pregnancy rate is 30% with crinone.

Non-inferiority margin is 10 percentage points (allows viable pregnancy rate down to 20% using prolutex).

This margin appears too big because if a pregnancy is lost there is no salvage therapy (<5 percentage point difference seems preferable).

Figure 5.5 Examples of non-inferiority margins in three disorders. Sources: Fleischmann *et al.*[30]; Swindells *et al.*[31]; Lockwood *et al*[32] Note that for the rheumatoid arthritis example,[30] switching *to* daily oral tablets is considered a key benefit for these particular patients (average age 50) to avoid frequent clinic visits. However, for the HIV example,[31] switching *from* daily tablets to a relatively infrequent single injection is the key benefit. It is important, therefore, to understand the circumstances and needs of different patient groups.

5.12 Multiplicity: multiple treatment arms or multiple outcome measures

When there are multiple intervention arms (≥3), investigators often wish to compare each pair, or certainly compare each new intervention with the control group. Multiple primary endpoints may feel appropriate for disorders with no obvious and well-established single endpoint. Also, if a new intervention can be effective for several 'major' outcome measures, this is likely to increase the strength of evidence making it more likely that decision-makers would recommend the new therapy. Some journals only allow the abstract of a clinical trial paper to refer to the single primary outcome measure, but if there are several major endpoints they are all expected to be included in the abstract particularly if they all show benefit.

The concept of multiplicity can apply to several primary endpoints, or one primary endpoint and several key secondary endpoints.[14, 33] It also allows investigators to have both hard and surrogate endpoints as major endpoints, instead of choosing one type.

Multiplicity increases the chance of finding spurious effects, such that the total error rate exceeds the generally accepted level of 5% (i.e. the more analyses performed, the more likely that a statistically significant result is observed but the finding is due to chance, e.g. the new treatment is not more effective/beneficial than the control). Various statistical methods can handle multiplicity, with the fundamental goal of keeping the overall error rate at 5% and maintaining the power of, for example, at least 80%. The term 'controlling the Family Wise Error Rate (FWER)' is used.

For multiple interventions, a **Bonferroni method** is a simple approach. If there are m treatment comparisons the error rate used in the sample size calculation would be $0.05/m$. Three possible comparisons exist with three treatment groups (e.g. two experimental and one standard therapy). The sample size error rate is now 0.017 (0.05/3). For example, to compare the proportions 50 versus 70% (80% power), 186 participants in total are needed using a 5% error rate, but this increases to 248 with 0.017% error rate. Also, statistical significance for interpreting the results is now defined as $p < 0.017$ (and not $p < 0.05$).

Attempts are made to distinguish *co-primary* from *multiple primary* endpoints, although there is no standard definition.

• Co-primary endpoints: *both* primary endpoints must be statistically significant to declare a 'positive' trial. Each endpoint is tested at a significance level of 0.05. Therefore, the study size can be the same as for one endpoint (0.05 used in the sample size calculation).

• Multiple primary endpoints: *any one* of the primary endpoints can be statistically significant to declare a 'positive' trial. Each endpoint is tested at a significance level determined by the method of multiplicity adjustment or simply by the partition of the significance (error) level. The study size is bigger than using a single primary endpoint because the error rates (significance levels) used for sample size are <0.05.

Box 5.6 Multiple endpoints: splitting *p*-values (see Figure 5.6) versus hierarchical testing

Splitting p-values	Typical gatekeeping (hierarchical) testing
Study size is bigger than using a single outcome	Study size can be the same as using a single outcome
Endpoints are considered separately	Endpoints have to be ranked (e.g. for clinical importance) upfront
Can claim an effect (benefit) for any endpoint on its own, regardless of the effects on other endpoints	A claim of effect for one endpoint depends on the results of the effects of all previous endpoints in the ranking (hierarchy)
Could analyse and report one endpoint before the others when the target number of patients and events have been achieved. E.g. in cancer trials progression-free survival could be published and submitted for an early regulatory license before overall survival.	All endpoints probably need to be analysed at the same time.

Simple and complex methods are available to handle multiple primary endpoints. Two common ways are **splitting or adjusting *p*-values** (e.g. the Bonferroni method) or **gatekeeping strategies** (referred to as **sequential or hierarchical testing**); Box 5.6.

Figure 5.6 is an example of splitting p-values to increase sample size. If study size is not increased, allowance for multiple outcomes can be made at the analysis stage using, for example Bonferroni or Hochberg approaches, or hierarchical testing (see Section 7.8, page 117).

5.13 Participants who switch trial interventions (crossover)

In surgical trials, for example, patients can change their mind after randomisation and request to have the procedure in the other group (**crossover**). These situations are sometimes unavoidable. Switching between trial interventions is also seen in trials of pharmaceutical medicines, especially when participants in one group who progress (do not respond) are then given the intervention for the other trial group. In drug trials,

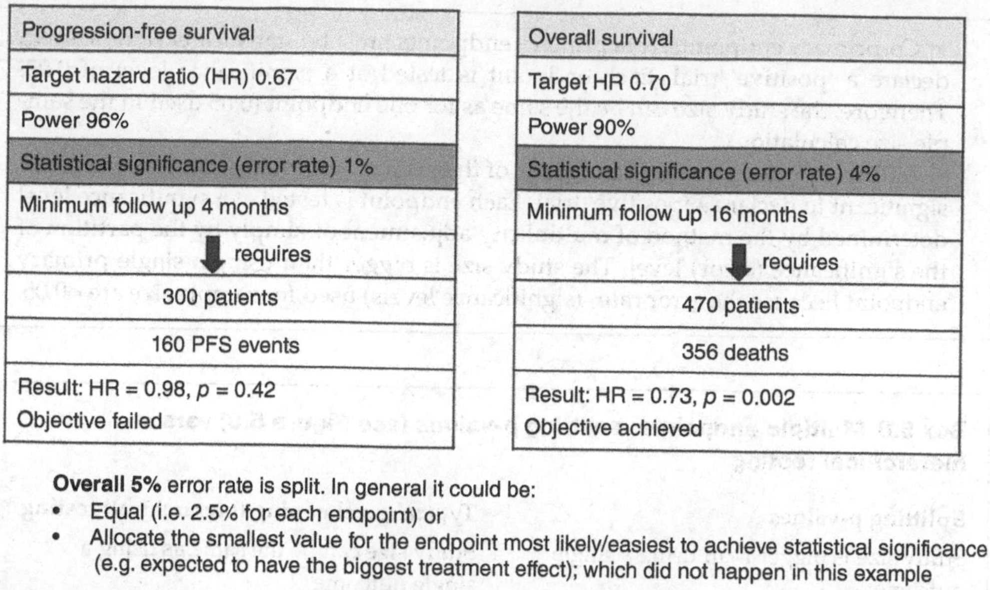

Progression-free survival
Target hazard ratio (HR) 0.67
Power 96%
Statistical significance (error rate) 1%
Minimum follow up 4 months
⬇ requires
300 patients
160 PFS events
Result: HR = 0.98, *p* = 0.42 Objective failed

Overall survival
Target HR 0.70
Power 90%
Statistical significance (error rate) 4%
Minimum follow up 16 months
⬇ requires
470 patients
356 deaths
Result: HR = 0.73, *p* = 0.002 Objective achieved

Overall 5% error rate is split. In general it could be:
- Equal (i.e. 2.5% for each endpoint) or
- Allocate the smallest value for the endpoint most likely/easiest to achieve statistical significance (e.g. expected to have the biggest treatment effect); which did not happen in this example

Figure 5.6 Illustration of splitting *p*-values across multiple primary endpoints (trial of second-line therapy pembrolizumab for advanced urothelial carcinoma).[34] If overall survival was the only primary endpoint, the required study size would be smaller, about 430 patients because of using 5% instead of 4% statistical significance.

the crossover is more likely to be patients in the control therapy group who are later given the experimental therapy when they progress, than vice versa. The main justification for doing so is to make the trial more appealing to health professionals and patients, because the controls could still (potentially) benefit from the experimental treatment. However, allowing crossover in the protocol can seriously impact the trial endpoints, leading to underestimation (dilution) of the treatment effect. An example is a trial of crizotinib versus standard chemotherapy for patients with advanced non-small cell lung cancer that have an ALK (anaplastic lymphoma kinase) gene mutation.[20] About 87% of patients who had chemotherapy (control arm) were allowed to switch to crizotinib, leading to no difference in overall survival. It essentially became a single-arm trial from which no reliable conclusion could be made about this endpoint.

It can be difficult to fully adjust the trial results for crossover, especially when there might be multiple (and unrecorded) reasons for it. Allowing crossover between the trial interventions should probably be avoided unless it has a clear scientific and ethical basis, and it does *not* affect major endpoints.

5.14 Summary points

- Phase III trials are considered the gold standard for evaluating a new intervention
- There are several designs, and all require specification of the new and control therapy, the randomisation process, outcome measures and follow-up schedule.
- There are several types of objectives: superiority, equivalence and non-inferiority.
- They should be sufficiently large to provide reliable evidence to change clinical practice.
- Designing non-inferiority and equivalence trials require careful consideration of the allowable margin.
- The main outcome measure(s) should be clinically relevant to the trial participants, researchers, health professionals and those who may benefit in the future.

References

1. US Food and Drug Administration. `https://www.fda.gov/regulatory-information/search-fda-guidance-documents/clinical-trials-guidance-documents`.
2. European Medicines Agency. `https://www.ema.europa.eu/en/human-regulatory/research-development/clinical-trials-human-medicines`.
3. Senn S. *Cross-over Trials in Clinical Research*. 2nd edn, John Wiley, 2002.
4. MRC Vitamin Study Research Group. Prevention of neural tube defects: results of the MRC vitamin study. *Lancet* 1991; **338**:132–137.
5. Pallmann P, Bedding AW, Choodari-Oskooei B *et al*. Adaptive designs in clinical trials: why use them, and how to run and report them. *BMC Med* 2018; **16**(1):29.
6. Park JJ, Thorlund K, Mills EJ. Critical concepts in adaptive clinical trials. *Clin Epidemiol* 2018; **10**:343–351.
7. Thorlund K, Haggstrom J, Park JJ *et al*. Key design considerations for adaptive clinical trials: a primer for clinicians. *BMJ* 2018; 360:k698. doi: `https://doi.org/10.1136/bmj.k698`.
8. Parmar MK, Barthel FM, Sydes M *et al*. Speeding up the evaluation of new agents in cancer. *J Natl Cancer Inst* 2008; **100**(17):1204–1214.
9. Park JJH, Hsu G, Siden EG *et al*. An overview of precision oncology basket and umbrella trials for clinicians. *CA Cancer J Clin* 2020; **70**(2):125–137.
10. Freidlin B, Korn EL. Biomarker enrichment strategies: matching trial design to biomarker credentials. *Nat Rev Clin Oncol* 2014; **11**(2):81–90.
11. Hemming K, Eldridge S, Forbes G *et al*. How to design efficient cluster randomised trials. *BMJ* 2017; **358**:j3064. doi: `https://doi.org/10.1136/bmj.j3064`.
12. Hemming K, Haines TP, Chilton PJ *et al*. The stepped wedge cluster randomised trial: rationale, design, analysis, and reporting. *BMJ* 2015; **350**:h391. doi: `https://doi.org/10.1136/bmj.h391`.
13. Govaert TME, Thijs CTMCN, Masurel N *et al*. The efficacy of influenza vaccination in elderly individuals. *JAMA* 1994; **272**(21):1661–1665.
14. Multiple Endpoints in Clinical Trials Guidance for Industry. Center for Drug Evaluation and Research (CDER). Food and Drug Administration. US Food and Drug Administration, January 2017. `https://www.fda.gov/files/drugs/published/Multiple-Endpoints-in-Clinical-Trials-Guidance-for-Industry.pdf`.
15. Montori VM, Permanyer-Miralda G, Ferreira-Goonzales I *et al*. Validity of composite end points in clinical trials. *BMJ* 2005; **330**:594–596.
16. Redfors B, Gregson J, Crowley A *et al*. The win ratio approach for composite endpoints: practical guidance based on previous experience. *Eur Heart J* 2020; **41**(46):4391–4399.
17. Ratitch B, Goel N, Mallinckrodt C *et al*. Defining efficacy estimands in clinical trials: examples illustrating ICH E9(R1) guidelines. *Ther Innov Regul Sci* 2020; **54**(2):370–384.
18. Ratitch B, Bell J, Mallinckrodt C *et al*. Choosing estimands in clinical trials: putting the ICH E9(R1) into practice. *Ther Innov Regul Sci* 2020; **54**(2):324–341.
19. Sticherling M, Mrowietz U, Augustin M *et al*. Secukinumab is superior to fumaric acid esters in treating patients with moderate-to-severe plaque psoriasis who are naive to systemic treatments: results from the randomized controlled PRIME trial. *Br J Dermatol* 2017; **177**(4):1024–1032.
20. Shaw AT, Kim DW, Nakagawa K *et al*. Crizotinib versus chemotherapy in advanced ALK-positive lung cancer. *N Engl J Med* 2013; **368**(25):2385–2394.
21. Machin D, Campbell M, Tan SB, Tan SH. *Sample Size Tables for Clinical Studies*. 3rd edn, Wiley-Blackwell Science, 2009 [comes with free software].
22. PS: Power and Sample size Calculation. `https://ps-power-and-sample-size-calculation.software.informer.com/3.1/`.
23. Southwest Oncology Group (SWOG). `https://stattools.crab.org/`
24. PASS (Power Analysis and Sample Size software): `http://www.ncss.com`.
25. nQuery. `http://www.statsols.com`.
26. Meurer WJ, Tolles J. Interim analyses during group sequential clinical trials. *JAMA* 2021; **326**(15):1524–1525.
27. Jones B, Jarvis P, Lewis JA, Ebbutt AF. Trials to assess equivalence: the importance of rigorous methods. *BMJ* 1996; 13:36–39.

28. Non-Inferiority Clinical Trials. Center for Drug Evaluation and Research (CDER). Food and Drug Administration. US Food and Drug Administration, November 2016. https://www.fda.gov/regulatory-information/search-fda-guidance-documents/non-inferiority-clinical-trials.

29. Guideline on the choice of the non-inferiority margin. European Medicines Agency. https://www.ema.europa.eu/en/documents/scientific-guideline/guideline-choice-non-inferiority-margin_en.pdf.

30. Fleischmann R, Mysler E, Hall S et al.; ORAL Strategy investigators. Efficacy and safety of tofacitinib monotherapy, tofacitinib with methotrexate, and adalimumab with methotrexate in patients with rheumatoid arthritis (ORAL Strategy): a phase 3b/4, double-blind, head-to-head, randomised controlled trial. *Lancet* 2017; **390**(10093):457–468.

31. Swindells S, Andrade-Villanueva JF, Richmond GJ et al. Long-acting Cabotegravir and Rilpivirine for maintenance of HIV-1 suppression. *N Engl J Med* 2020; **382**(12):1112–1123.

32. Lockwood G, Griesinger G, Cometti B; 13 European Centers. Subcutaneous progesterone versus vaginal progesterone gel for luteal phase support in in vitro fertilization: a noninferiority randomized controlled study. *Fertil Steril* 2014; **101**(1):112–119.

33. Vickerstaff V, Omar RZ, Ambler G. Methods to adjust for multiple comparisons in the analysis and sample size calculation of randomised controlled trials with multiple primary outcomes. *BMC Med Res Methodol* 2019; **19**(1):129.

34. Bellmunt J, de Wit R, Vaughn DJ et al.; KEYNOTE-045 Investigators. Pembrolizumab as Second-Line Therapy for Advanced Urothelial Carcinoma. *N Engl J Med* 2017; 376(11):1015–1026.

CHAPTER 6

Phase III trials – fundamental aspects of analysis and interpretation

Randomised controlled phase III trials usually aim to change practice, so their data need careful analysis and appropriate interpretation. Several textbooks provide details on methods of analyses.[1,2] Figure 1.1 (page 2) and Box 2.1 (page 16) outline the main outcome measures that should be reported. This chapter provides an overview of common aspects of analysis and interpretation:

- efficacy (for each of the three fundamental categories of endpoints), along with confidence intervals and p-values/statistical significance
- adverse events
- adherence
- health-related quality of life (QoL)
- intention-to-treat and per protocol analyses.

Many of these concepts can also apply to phase I and II trials. Although the different categories of outcomes are reported separately (efficacy, safety, adherence and QoL), the overall benefit-harm balance needs to be assessed. This is not often easy to do and it can be worthwhile involving patient/public representatives. Also, the relative importance of each type of outcome might depend on the disorder and intervention. For example, exercise and diet for chronic disorders/symptoms should have minimal side effects hence there could be more attention to QoL. Whereas for fatal disorders, some patients may view QoL as less important than efficacy.

6.1 Efficacy

An **effect size**# is a single *quantitative* summary measure used to interpret clinical trial data and help communicate the results to health professionals and the public/patients. It is obtained by comparing a trial outcome measure between two intervention groups.

Interpreting effect sizes:
- Is there a difference (effect) and how big is it?
- What is the **clinical importance/relevance** of the result?
- What could the true effect size be (**95% confidence interval**)?
- Could the observed effect be a chance finding in this particular trial (*p***-value/statistical significance**)?

There is another use of this term which is the standardized difference (Section 'Outcome measures based on taking measurements on people'), but in this book the general term is used.

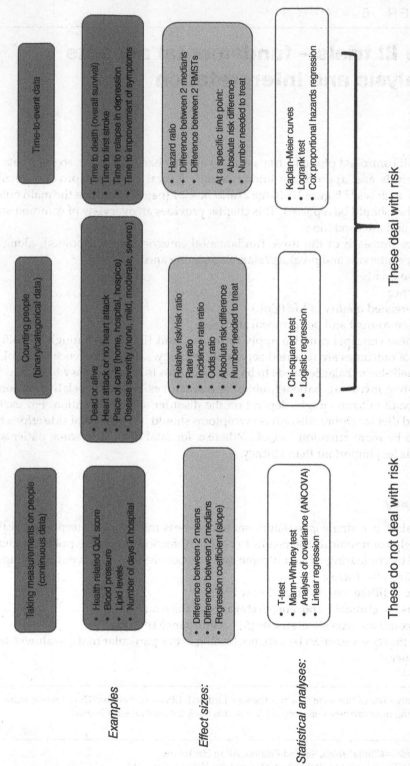

Figure 6.1 Overview of the three fundamental categories of outcome measures, and corresponding effect sizes and common statistical analyses. QoL, quality of life; RMST, restricted mean survival time. 'Risk' used generally to reflect chance, odds, likelihood, or hazard for a person to have an event.

Researchers often have the impression that there are many different effect sizes to choose from, but once the type of outcome measure is understood there are a limited number of effect sizes (Figure 6.1). The type of outcome measure determines how the study size is estimated, the method of statistical analysis, and the interpretation of the trial. Some effect sizes can be calculated by hand, and others require statistical software.

When interpreting the results, investigators should see whether the trial participants were representative of the target population (generalisable), because the efficacy and adverse event profiles could be influenced by this.

Outcome measures based on counting people

Consider a trial that evaluated the effect of giving an influenza vaccine to the elderly (Box 6.1).[3]

What are the main results?

Each percentage (or proportion) indicates the **risk** (chance) of developing flu. For example, the risk of being diagnosed with flu by serology after 5 months in the placebo arm is 8.8%. The two percentages are combined into a single **effect size**: either the ratio (**relative risk** or **risk ratio**) or difference (**absolute risk difference** or **absolute risk reduction** [**ARR**]) – Figure 6.2. The **comparison** or **reference group** must always be made clear, and noted whether it is new therapy versus control, or vice versa, as the interpretation depends on the ordering. We now interpret the clinical implications of these results (Box 6.2). Some interventions have such obviously large effects that everyone agrees. Different interpretations tend to arise for moderate and especially small effects.

**Box 6.1 Example: Phase III trial of the influenza vaccine in the elderly.
Source: Govaert et al.[3]**

Location: 15 family health practices in the Netherlands

Participants: 1838 men and women aged ≥60 years

Intervention: Single flu vaccine injection

Control: Single placebo (saline) injection (hence a double-blind placebo-controlled trial)

Outcome measure: The proportion who developed flu up to 5 months after the injection; diagnosed by (i) serology or (ii) family doctor

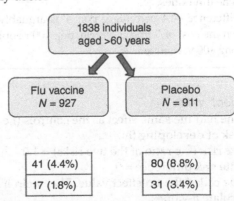

Flu diagnosis 5 months later	Flu vaccine N = 927	Placebo N = 911
By serology	41 (4.4%)	80 (8.8%)
By family doctor	17 (1.8%)	31 (3.4%)

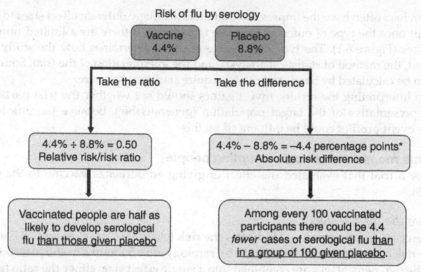

Figure 6.2 Turning two percentages (risks) into a single effect size. For the risk difference, the minus sign just indicates fewer events.* 'Percentage points' is used instead of the symbol '%' to avoid confusion with another effect size that uses %.

Box 6.2 Is the effect size a small, moderate or big effect?

This is a fairly crude categorization to start thinking about clinical importance, and we generally consider:

1. What is being prevented or treated (how serious is the disorder)?
2. How big is the benefit (the quantitative effect size)?
3. How common is the disorder?

We may also consider adverse events, quality of life and costs.

Interpreting the treatment effect depends on the type of effect size used. People's interpretation of the same effect size will often vary, and also depend on the point of view from the patient/public, health professional or the healthcare provider (payer).

• In the flu vaccine trial, 'Relative risk 0.5' is a **big effect**. Not many interventions can halve the risk of a disorder, and influenza is a common disorder in the elderly that can lead to serious health issues.

• 'Risk difference −4.4 percentage points' is arguably a **moderate effect** (some might say small given the cost of/effort in vaccinating 100 people), since this represents only 4 fewer cases among 100 vaccinated.

The 'no-effect' value

If the vaccine had the same effect as the controls (i.e. no effect), both groups would have the same risk of developing flu:

• Relative risk (the ratio of the two risks) = 1.0
• Absolute risk difference = 0

These can be called the no-effect value. They help interpret confidence intervals and are used to calculate *p*-values.

Is the new intervention better or worse?

Relative risk, risk ratio or risk difference indicates the magnitude of the effect. Determining whether the intervention is more beneficial or harmful depends on what is measured. 'Risk' implies something bad, but in research, it can be used for any endpoint. If the outcome measure is 'positive', for example, the percentage of people who are alive, or the percentage of patients with psoriasis whose symptoms have improved, an <u>increased</u> relative risk (i.e. >1), or <u>positive</u> risk difference (i.e. >0), indicates that the new intervention is more beneficial. If the outcome measure is 'negative', such as the percentage of people who have died, or the percentage of patients with psoriasis whose quality of life has deteriorated, a <u>decreased</u> relative risk (i.e. <1) or <u>negative</u> risk difference indicates that the new intervention is more beneficial.

Converting relative risks

Relative risks of 0.5 or 2.0 are easy to interpret: the risk is half or twice as large as in the reference group. Alternatively, they can be converted to a **percentage change in risk**: either a **relative risk reduction** or an **excess risk**. Using Box 6.1, the relative risk of clinician-diagnosed flu is 0.53 (1.8/3.4%). The percentage change in risk is found simply by subtracting the relative risk from 1.0 (the no effect value) then multiplying by 100. So the risk of flu is reduced by 47% in those who were vaccinated, compared with placebo. Similarly, a relative risk of 1.87, for example, represents an 87% increase in risk. Generally, relative risks below 2.0 can be converted, while those above 2.0 are left alone to avoid looking cumbersome (e.g., a relative risk of 12 is an 1100% excess risk).

Number Needed to Treat (NNT)

NNT is just another way of expressing absolute risk difference. The risk difference for serological flu is −4.4 percentage points:

Among 100 vaccinated participants, there were 4.4 fewer cases of serological flu (compared to placebo)

Among 23 (100/4.4) vaccinated participants there was 1 (4.4/4.4) less case of flu

NNT: to avoid one case of serological flu, 23 people need to be vaccinated (treated)

NNT sometimes has intuitive appeal, but there are limitations.[4] It can be specific to the characteristics of the trial participants. Importantly, it can change over time, with more follow-up and more events. Nevertheless, NNT might be useful for comparing between different interventions or disorders, acknowledging that it may not reflect the clinical importance of each disorder.

Relative or absolute effects?

Both are useful. Relative effects (the ratio of two summary statistics) such as relative risk tend to be similar across different populations (but not always), indicating the effect of a new intervention *generally*. They do not usually depend on the underlying (background) rate of a disorder. A relative risk of 0.5 means that the risk is halved from whatever it is in a particular population, whether the usual flu incidence is 1 per 100 or 20 per 100. However, absolute effects (the difference between two summary statistics) such as risk difference always reflect the underlying rate, and so will vary between populations. It indicates the *impact* of an intervention *in a particular population*. Table 6.1 illustrates this.

Table 6.1 Relative risk and risk difference according to different underlying disease rates (the placebo group). As the background risk gets higher, the relative risk remains the same (i.e. a halving of risk is a big effect), but the risk difference and NNT go from a small to large effect.

Risk of flu				
Placebo (background) (per 100)	*Vaccine (per 100)*	*Relative risk*	*Absolute risk difference (per 1000)*	*The number needed to treat to avoid one event*
1	0.5	0.50	5 (small effect)	200
2	1.0	0.50	10	100
5	2.5	0.50	25	40
10	5.0	0.50	50	20
20	10.0	0.50	100 (large effect)	10

Odds ratio versus relative risk

Sometimes, an **odds ratio** is reported instead of relative risk. 'Risk' and 'odds' are different ways of presenting the likelihood of having a disorder. Risk is the number with disease out of all participants, while odds expresses the number with disease to the number without. If there is one affected person among n people, the risk value is $1/n$ while the odds are $1/(n-1)$, or $1: n-1$.

For fairly uncommon disorders (e.g. <20%), relative risk and odds ratio are often similar, and so can be *interpreted* in the same way (Table 6.2A). However, when the disorder is common, they will be noticeably different (Table 6.2B). A ratio of two odds is not the same as a ratio of two risks. In Table 6.2B, it would be incorrect to interpret the odds ratio of 0.25 as a risk reduction of 75%. The risk has been reduced by 51%,

Table 6.2 Calculation of relative risk and odds ratio using the flu vaccine trial (serological diagnosis).

(A) Incidence of flu is uncommon (from the trial in Box 6.1)

	Developed flu	*Did not develop flu*	*Total*
Vaccine group	41 (a)	886 (b)	927 (n_1)
Placebo group	80 (c)	831 (d)	911 (n_2)

Relative risk = $a/n_1 \div c/n_2$ (41/927) ÷ (80/911) = 0.50
Odds of developing flu in the vaccine group = 41/886 (a/b)
Odds of developing flu in the placebo group = 80/831 (c/d)
Odds ratio is (41/886) ÷ (80/831) = (a × d) ÷ (c × b) = 0.48

(B) Incidence of flu is common (hypothetical results)

	Developed flu	*Did not develop flu*	*Total*
Vaccine group	300	627	927
Placebo group	600	311	911

Relative risk = (300/927) ÷ (600/911) = 0.49
Odds ratio = (300 × 311) ÷ (627 × 600) = 0.25

indicated by the relative risk of 0.49, but the odds in the vaccine group are 0.25 times the odds in the placebo group. This is difficult to explain easily. When a disorder is common, describing an odds ratio as if it were a relative risk could overestimate the treatment effect; relative risk may be preferable. The odds ratio has mathematical properties that form the basis of standard statistical methods (e.g. logistic regression), which is why it is often used.

Incidence rate ratio

The denominators for relative risk and odds ratio are based on the number of participants in a trial group, which is acceptable when participants have similar lengths of follow-up or the concept of follow-up does not apply. When follow-up times vary, one approach is to use methods for time-to-event data (Section 'Outcome measures based on time-to-event data' on page 88). An alternative simple method is to use **person-years**. This allows for different exposure times to an intervention or different lengths of time during which events (e.g. deaths or occurrence of a disorder) can occur:

Participant number 1 followed up for 5.3 years
Participant number 2 followed up for 2.8 years
Together, these two people have 8.1 person-years.

An incidence rate (measure of risk) is the number of people with an event (numerator) divided by the total number of person-years (denominator). For example, New Treatment (28 deaths out of 13,218 person-years) ÷ Controls (39 deaths out of 12,548 person-years), is an incidence rate ratio of 0.68. The incidence rate (e.g. likelihood of dying) is reduced by 32% using the new therapy compared with the controls (a similar interpretation to relative risk, but incidence rate is technically not the same as risk where the denominator is the number of people).

Outcome measures based on taking measurements on people

Here, the trial endpoint in each arm is often summarised by the mean value and the standard deviation (Chapter 2). It can apply to a wide range of endpoints, including physical and physiological measures (e.g. body weight and blood pressure), biomarkers (e.g. lipid levels), and psychological measures (e.g. depression scores). This section shows simple ways to analyse and interpret this type of outcome measure. Other approaches are provided in Section 6.4 (that covers health-related quality of life) and in Chapter 7 (repeated measures analysis). An appropriate effect size is the **difference between two means** (or **mean difference**), if the data follow a Normal/Gaussian (symmetric) distribution, so simple statistical analyses can be used. Otherwise, **difference between the two medians** is often better for skewed (asymmetric) distributions.

What are the main results?

Box 6.3 shows an example where the primary trial endpoint is body weight.[5] With 'taking measurements on people' endpoints, the baseline value is usually allowed for because this naturally varies between participants. Obtaining the mean difference can be done in two common ways:

1. For each person, take their weight at 12 months minus weight at baseline (i.e. the change), then calculate the mean value of the change for each trial group. The mean difference is then Mean Change$_{\text{low-fat}}$ minus Mean Change$_{\text{low-carbohydrate}}$. This is acceptable if the baseline values are similar between the trial groups.

2. Perform a **multivariable linear regression analysis** where weight at 12 months is the 'outcome variable', and the baseline weight and treatment groups are 'covariates'. This analysis produces the mean difference in body weight at 12 months between the trial arms, after allowing for each person's baseline value.[6, 7] The mean difference obtained from regression models can be called **Least Squares means (LS means),** or **placebo-corrected LS means** (if the control arm is a placebo). They are often adjusted for several baseline factors.

The mean difference calculated using either of the above approaches is sometimes similar.

At 12 months, the low-fat diet group lost an average of 5.29 kg from baseline, compared with 5.99 kg in the low-carbohydrate diet group. The effect size (**mean difference**) is 0.70 kg: the low-fat diet group gained an average of 0.7 kg *more* than the low-carbohydrate diet group. But this is a small clinical effect (using Box 6.2).

The effect size is associated with an *average* difference in weight change; this single number cannot represent all trial participants. In each diet group, individuals would have lost weight, gained weight or had no weight change. It is always worth seeing the individual values (particularly to look for outliers that might be of biological interest). This is shown in Figure 6.3, which is a scatterplot where many people lost weight, but the pattern is similar between the trial groups. An alternative is a waterfall plot (see Figure 3.5 page 38 as an example).

Understanding the clinical effect in Box 6.3 is easy because everyone is familiar with body weight and kilograms. However, for other continuous measures (e.g. depression or pain scores), the unit of measurement is not as obvious so additional information is needed:

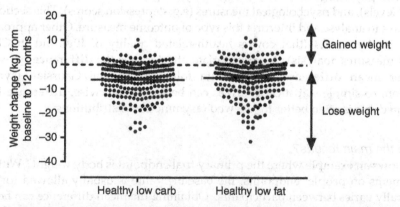

Figure 6.3 Scatter plot showing the weight change for each trial participant using the example in Box 6.3 (horizontal lines indicate the mean change). The figure was produced using approximate data points taken from the original figure (waterfall plot).[5]

Box 6.3 Example: Phase III trial comparing two diets. Source: Gardner et al.[5]

Location: Stanford and San Francisco (California, US)

Participants: 609 men and women aged 18–50 years with body mass index 28–40 kg/m^2

Intervention: Healthy low-fat diet for 1 year (dietary instructions via 22 group sessions)

Control: Healthy low-carbohydrate diet for 1 year (dietary instructions via 22 group sessions)

Outcome measure: Change in body weight (from baseline to 12 months after starting the diet)

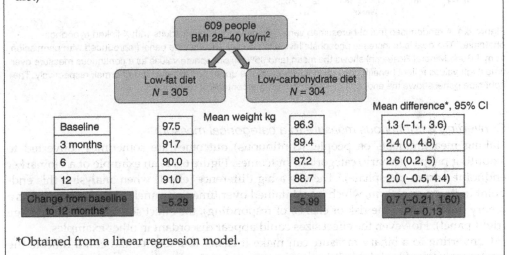

	Mean weight kg		Mean difference*, 95% CI
Baseline	97.5	96.3	1.3 (–1.1, 3.6)
3 months	91.7	89.4	2.4 (0, 4.8)
6	90.0	87.2	2.6 (0.2, 5)
12	91.0	88.7	2.0 (–0.5, 4.4)
Change from baseline to 12 months*	–5.29	–5.99	0.7 (–0.21, 1.60) P = 0.13

*Obtained from a linear regression model.

- the scale (range) of the measurement
- whether a high value reflects benefit or harm
- whether there exists a minimum clinically important difference (often determined by those who created the measurement, e.g. quality of life scales).

This is covered in more detail in Section 6.4 (quality of life, see Figure 6.10).

Some investigators calculate a **standardised mean difference** as the effect size (can be called **Cohen's d**), which is the difference between two means divided by the standard deviation (SD) of the difference. This standardises the outcome such that the unit of measurement is no longer the original scale but rather the number of SD units. Values around 0.2, 0.4 and above 0.7 broadly represent small, moderate and large effects, respectively.

Another way is to express the difference between the two means as a percentage change (e.g. if the mean body weight is 105 kg with Diet A and 118 kg with Diet B, there is an 11% reduction in weight with Diet A [105 – 118/118]). This might make the results easier to interpret and communicate but can overestimate the effect sometimes.

The 'no-effect' value

If the low-fat diet had no effect compared to the low-carbohydrate diet, both groups would have the same change in body weight. The mean difference is then zero.

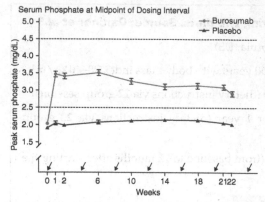

	Burosumab N = 68	Placebo N = 66
% (number) who responded*	94.1% (64)	7.6% (5)
Relative risk	12.4 (94.1÷7.6)	
Absolute risk difference	86.5 percentage points (94.1–7.6)	

*Each patient's phosphate values are averaged over time; the patient is a 'responder' if this is greater than the lower limit for normal.

Figure 6.4 A randomised trial of burosumab versus placebo for treating adults with X-linked hypophos-phatemia.[8] The goal is to increase phosphate levels to normal. The left side panel (reproduced with permission from J Bone Mineral Research) shows the mean (and 95%CI) phosphate values as a continuous measure over time (high values reflect benefit); the horizontal lines are the upper and lower limit for normal, respectively. The right side panel shows the endpoint converted to risk (percentage of responders).

Converting a continuous measure to a categorical measure

'Taking measurements on people' (continuous) outcomes are sometimes converted to 'counting people' (binary/categorical) outcomes. Figure 6.4 is an example of a biomarker endpoint (serum phosphate).[8] There is a big difference (effect) when analysing this end-point in its original form, which is maintained over time (left panel). When expressed as a binary outcome (i.e. the risk or chance of responding), the effect sizes are also very large (right panel). However, the effect sizes could appear discordant in other examples.

Converting to a binary measure can make it easier to interpret and communicate the treatment effect. Also, highlighting an extreme end of the distribution of the measurement might be more clinically relevant. However, the use of risk ignores variability in the measurement (i.e. a less sensitive analysis), and there is often less statistical power (more participants are needed to show statistical significance).

Outcome measures based on time-to-event data
What are the main results?

Box 6.4 is an example.[9] The event of interest is death from any cause. The Kaplan–Meier curves are shown in Figure 6.5. The full y-axis is 0–100%. Truncated plots (e.g. y-axis 0 to 20%) can magnify treatment effects, making them appear larger than they really are.

The length of median follow-up can be obtained using Kaplan-Meier curves (e.g. people who have died are censored at their death date, and those still alive have their last known date treated as an event date).

The number of patients at risk at the bottom is important. This decreases over time because people either have an event (here, died) or are censored (see Section 2.6 page 22 for reasons for censoring). The numbers at risk reflect the reliability of the curve. With very few participants at risk (e.g. <10, after month 30), that part of the curve is unreliable, so comparisons at those time points should be avoided. With longer follow-up, someone initially censored at 12 months could then appear at 24 months, and the numbers at risk will change.

If participants given the new therapy are more likely than the controls to be censored before they have the event of interest (e.g. censored when they stop treatment due to

Box 6.4 Example: Phase III trial of avelumab for treating cancer. Source: Powles et al.[9]

Location: 197 centres in 2 countries.

Participants: 700 patients with unresectable advanced urothelial cancer who had already completed first-line chemotherapy and whose disease had not progressed.

Intervention: Avelumab given as maintenance therapy (intravenously every 2 weeks) plus best supportive care (BSC)

Control: BSC only

Outcome measure: Overall survival (time to death from any cause); patients alive were censored at the date of last contract.

[BSC: any therapy considered appropriate for the patient, and palliative care including radiotherapy; but other systemic anti-cancer drugs were not allowed].

Use vertical line to get event rates (proportions) at a time point
(read off *y*-axis): 71.3 vs 58.4%

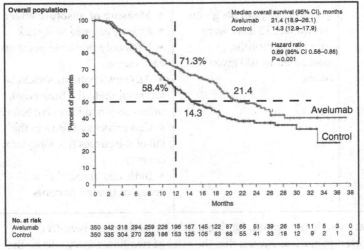

Use horizontal line to get median times (read off *x*-axis): 21.4 vs 14.3 months

Figure 6.5 Overall survival curves for the trial in Box 6.4. Three effect sizes can be obtained: hazard ratio, the difference in median survival, and absolute risk difference (at 12 months); Box 6.5. Source: Powles et al.[9]/figure reproduced with permission from the Massachusetts Medical Society/NEJM.

having an adverse event), this could make the new treatment appear to be more effective than it really is (**informative censoring**). This is because events that occur after censoring are not recorded or counted in the new treatment group, and having fewer events compared to the control therapy could contribute to the appearance of improved benefit. To avoid this, all participants should be followed up as much as possible.

For superiority trials, the bigger the gap between the Kaplan–Meier curves, the larger the treatment effect. Several effect sizes can be obtained, and they each tell us something different about the comparison of the trial treatments (Box 6.5). The difference in median

Box 6.5 Three effect sizes for time-to-event data using the trial in Box 6.4 and Figure 6.5.[9] Considering whether the treatment has a small, moderate or big effect depends on which effect size is interpreted (see also Box 6.2)

Effect size	Interpretation	Comments
Hazard ratio 0.69[#]	The risk (hazard) of dying is decreased by 31% using avelumab (at any single time point; having survived to that time)	• **Measure of relative effect** • *Efficacy assessed using risk* • Uses the whole Kaplan–Meier curve • Assumes proportional hazards*
Difference in median: Median OS (21.4 – 14.3 months = 7.1)	Patients given avelumab were alive, on average[#], 7.1 months longer than those on BSC alone (median OS is 7.1 months longer)	• **Measure of absolute effect** • *Efficacy assessed using time* • Uses only one point on each curve (can be influenced by chance) • Easy for patients and clinicians to understand
Absolute risk difference: 12-month OS rate (71.3% – 58.4% = 13 percentage points)	Among 100 patients given avelumab, 13 *more* were alive at 12 months, compared to 100 given BSC alone	• **Measure of absolute effect** • *Efficacy assessed using risk* • Uses only one time point on each curve • All (most) patients should be followed up to the time point, unless they had the event before • Can reflect a plateau in the tail of the curves (i.e. long-term benefit) • Indicates 'impact' in a group of treated patients

*The risk of an event at a single time point, having reached that time as event-free, is called a hazard. Proportional hazards means that the ratio of two hazards should be the same at all time points (except at the very start). #'average' is used informally, and the difference in median cannot reflect the benefit in all participants. OS: overall survival. BSC: best supportive care.

times should be interpreted in context with the control value (e.g. a difference of 6 months is a big effect when the control median is 2 months, but perhaps a small effect when the control value is 10 years). Sometimes two medians are expressed as a relative effect (e.g. an improvement from 10 to 15 months is a 50% increase). This is acceptable but note that

[#] Compares two Kaplan-Meier curves, as a relative effect (imagine it as dividing one curve by the other). If two therapies have the same effect, the curves will overlap completely, so the hazard ratio will be 1.0.

improving the median from 1 to 1.5 weeks has the same 50% increase as 10 to 15 months, yet they represent very different impacts (value) to individuals.

For harmful events such as death or disease occurrence, a hazard ratio (HR) <1 means that the new intervention is more beneficial than the control because the risk of having an event is reduced (i.e. participants have taken longer to develop the event). But for 'good' events such as disease has disappeared, the ability to function or symptoms improve, a HR >1 indicates benefit.

In the example, the absolute risk difference of 13 percentage points was obtained using the two observed proportions at 12 months. A more reliable estimate of the risk difference could be calculated using the event rate in the control arm and the hazard ratio:

12-month OS rate in the control arm $(P) = 0.584$ (58.4%)

Hazard ratio (HR) = 0.69

Risk difference in 12-month PFS proportion (avelumab – control) = $e^{HR \times \log_e P} - P$

= $e^{0.69 \times \log_e 0.584} - 0.584 = 0.11$ (11 percentage points)$^#$

The 95%CI for the difference can be obtained easily by substituting the 95%CI limits for the HR into the above formula.

It is worth comparing HR (time-to-event endpoints) and relative risk ('counting people' endpoints). Both are measures of the likelihood of having an event, but relative risk ignores time per participant (it just uses the total number of events at the end of the study), but HR allows for time per participant (i.e. time for an event to occur or follow-up time for people who did not have an event). Although HR is sometimes expressed as a reduction or increase in risk, because this is easier to explain, technically it is the hazard that changes (not risk). The word 'risk' therefore has a broader meaning than its technical definition when interpreting hazard ratios.

The 'no-effect' value

If two interventions have the same effect their Kaplan-Meier curves would completely overlap. Hence, the no effect value for the HR would be 1.0, while the no effect value for the absolute risk difference would be 0.

Relative or absolute effects?

As with 'counting people endpoints', both relative and absolute effects are useful. Consider a trial of erlotinib versus placebo for treating advanced pancreatic cancer,[10] with overall survival (time to death from any cause) as the primary endpoint. The HR of 0.81 ($p = 0.03$) indicated a moderate 19% reduction in the risk (hazard) of dying. However, the median survival was 6.37 months with erlotinib and 5.95 months with placebo: a benefit of only 2 weeks, which is a very small effect, especially given the side effects and drug cost. This example illustrates clearly that the interpretation of a treatment effect depends on which type of effect size is used (see also Box 6.2).

Number needed to treat

Absolute risk difference and NNT using time-to-event outcomes have the same interpretation as that for 'counting people' endpoints (page 83) but for time-to-event outcomes they must be linked to a time point. Figure 6.6 is an example showing that both of these effect sizes change over time.

$^#$ 'e' is the exponential constant (2.71828), also known as Euler's number.

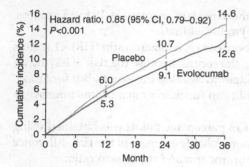

Month	Risk (%)	Absolute risk difference (percentage points)	NNT
12	5.3 vs 6.0	−0.7	143
24	9.1 vs 10.7	−1.6	62.5
36	12.6 vs 14.6	−2.0	50

Figure 6.6 Illustration of how absolute risk difference and number needed to treat (NNT) can change over time, using a trial of evolocumab versus placebo for patients with atherosclerotic cardiovascular disease (composite primary endpoint is the cumulative incidence of cardiovascular death, myocardial infarction, stroke, hospitalisation for unstable angina, or coronary revascularisation). Source: Sabatine et al.[11]/figure reproduced with permission from the Massachusetts Medical Society/NEJM.

Alternative to the hazard ratio

HR assumes that the treatment relative effect is similar over time, e.g. the ratio of the hazards at 2 years is the same as at 4 years (assumption of proportional hazards, and there is a statistical test to check this). This assumption is violated when, for example, the Kaplan-Meier curves clearly cross over each other (e.g. see Figure 7.8a, page 122), or they overlap for some time and only separate later on (or vice versa). HRs are still reported because people expect them. They are sometimes said to represent an 'average' effect over time, but they need to be interpreted with caution because a single hazard ratio cannot reflect how the treatment effect varies over time. Alternatively, the absolute risk difference at two or more pre-specified time points (e.g. early and late) could be interpreted.

Another approach is to use **restricted mean survival time** (RMST) which uses the whole Kaplan-Meier curve. This is the area under the curve. An RMST for a curve based on overall survival is a measure of the average duration of survival over the full follow-up period (sometimes labelled life expectancy). RMSTs can be used regardless of the shape of the Kaplan-Meier curves and there is no assumption of proportional hazards. Life expectancy difference and ratio (LED and LER) are simple absolute and relative effect sizes, respectively.[12]

What could the true effect size be (confidence intervals)?

95% Confidence Interval for any effect size

A range within which the **true** effect size* is expected to lie with a high degree of certainty.

If we conducted 100 similar trials, each producing a confidence interval, we expect 95 to contain the true value of the effect size and 5 would not just by chance.

*Relative risk, odds ratio, hazards ratio, absolute risk difference, mean difference, etc.

When we conduct a clinical trial, we aim to estimate the **true** effect of a new intervention. It can be thought of as the effect among all participants who could benefit from the therapy now and in the future. There is always uncertainty over how close the observed effect size from a trial will be to the true effect size. This is quantified by a **standard error**, used to calculate a **95% confidence interval** for an effect size (standard formulae can be used, and there are free web-based calculators). The basic principle is the same as that for a single proportion or mean (Chapter 4):

95% CI for a true effect size = observed effect size ± 1.96 × standard error of the effect size

From the example in Box 6.1 (flu vaccine trial), the observed relative risk was 0.50, and the 95%CI is calculated to be 0.35 to 0.72. Although our best estimate of the **true** relative risk is 0.50, we consider that the true effect is highly likely to be somewhere between 0.35 and 0.72.* Importantly, this interval *excludes* the no-effect value (relative risk of 1.0), hence a real effect is likely. In general, for superiority trials we wish to see:

- Narrow confidence interval (CI), indicating precise (reliable) results
- CI that does not overlap (include) the no-effect value
- CI that is far from the no-effect value, if the new treatment really has a big effect

---

Describing a CI sometimes implies that the true effect size lies anywhere within the range with the same likelihood. However, the true effect is more likely to be close to the point estimate used to derive the interval (i.e. the middle) than at the extreme ends.[13] This is an important consideration when the interval just overlaps the no-effect value. With a relative risk of 0.75, and 95% CI 0.55–1.03, most of the range is below the no-effect value. Although the possibility of 'no effect' cannot be reliably excluded, a treatment effect should not be dismissed because there is a clear suggestion of a benefit.[13]

Could the observed effect size be a chance finding (p-values and statistical significance)?

In the flu vaccine trial (Box 6.1), the observed risk difference associated with serological flu was −4.4 percentage points. A question we ask is:

Could the observed difference −4.4 percentage points be a chance (lucky/spurious) finding in this particular trial?

The answer to this question (and for any trial and any disorder) is always strictly YES.

P-values allow us to quantify this.

The *p*-value for the risk difference of −4.4 percentage points, where each risk was based on 41/927 and 80/911, is calculated to be <0.001. If there really were no effect of the flu vaccine (i.e. the true difference were zero), a value of −4.4 percentage points could be seen in some studies, just by chance. But how often?

The *p*-value of <0.001 indicates that a difference as large as 4.4 or greater could occur in less than 1 in 1000 studies of a similar size and design by chance alone, *assuming* that the vaccine had the same effect as placebo. The observed effect size is "*unlikely to have arisen*

---

* Although this is not the strict definition of CI, little is lost by this description for practical use. If confidence intervals were calculated from many different studies of a similar size and design, 95% of them should contain the true value.

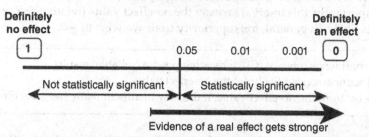

- *P*-values lie on a continuous scale
- They address the question
'*Could the observed effect size from the trial be a chance/lucky/spurious finding?*'

Definition: The probability that an effect size as large as that observed, or more extreme, is due to chance **if there really were no effect**

All p-values are between 0 and 1

Definitely no effect

Definitely an effect

1   0.05   0.01   0.001   0

Not statistically significant   Statistically significant

Evidence of a real effect gets stronger

Figure 6.7 P-values. Those for superiority trials *assume* there is really (truly) no effect; a different assumption is made for non-inferiority trials (see Chapter 7). In general, *p*-values larger than 0.01 should be shown to two decimal places, those between 0.01 and 0.001 to three decimal places, and those smaller than 0.001 could be shown as $p < 0.001$. They should not be reported as '<0.05' or '≥0.05' because this is too crude.

by chance" and we simplify this and conclude "*there is a real effect of the vaccine*". Our conclusion could be wrong but only 1 in 1000 times; a *p*-value is an error rate.

The $p < 0.001$ is actually a **two-tailed** *p*-value. Effect sizes of −4.4 percentage points or lower (vaccine better than placebo), or +4.4 percentage points or greater (placebo better than vaccine), are both plausible. Therefore, any departure from the no-effect value in either extreme direction is allowed for. The *p*-value is twice as large as a **one-tailed** *p*-value, which is based on looking only in a single direction. The more conservative two-tailed *p*-value is reported for most trials, unless a one-tailed value can be properly justified (i.e. the new treatment can only be better).

Figure 6.7 shows the definition of *p*-values. A new intervention is considered to have a real effect if the *p*-value is <0.05: the result is said to be **statistically significant**. *P*-values >0.05 indicate that the result is **not statistically significant**, so there is insufficient evidence of a real effect. The size of a p-value is determined by two components (Figure 6.8).

> Researchers should always distinguish **clinical importance** (effect size is small, moderate or big, and the benefit/impact for people, see Box 6.2) from **statistical significance** (which addresses one specific question about the study result and the influence of chance).

Misinterpretation of p-values

There is nothing scientific about the cut-off of 0.05 when determining statistical significance. It was initially recommended as a *guideline* for making decisions, but it has become a fixed rule instead. 'Statistically significant' for $p < 0.05$ and 'not statistically significant' for $p \geq 0.05$ have unfortunately become synonymous with 'there is a real treatment effect' and 'there is no effect' respectively. But if the effect size looks clinically meaningful (e.g. relative risk 0.60), it is absurd to conclude the treatment is effective

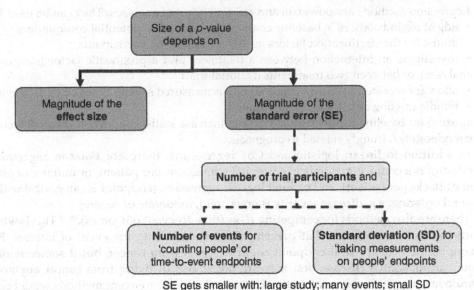

SE gets smaller with: large study; many events; small SD

Small p-values arise from: big effect size, big study, many events, or small SD

Figure 6.8 What determines the size of a *p*-value.

if $p = 0.049$ but ineffective if $p = 0.051$ because they provide practically the same level of evidence. Yet a stark difference in conclusions is often made. Clinical trial experts have discussed this problem.[13-17] Careful interpretation is needed when *p*-values are just above 0.05 (Box 6.6). If an effect size is not statistically significant, it means that there is insufficient evidence to claim an effect, and there are several reasons:

1. There really is no effect (new therapy has same effect as controls)
2. There is a real effect, but by chance the sample of participants did not show this
3. There is a real effect which is seen in the trial, but there is **insufficient power** (too few participants or events), to detect it reliably and make $p < 0.05$ (see also Figure 6.8).

How are effect sizes, confidence intervals and *p*-values obtained?

They come from performing a **statistical test/analysis**.[1, 2] The choice of test depends on the type of outcome measure. Figure 6.1 shows some common statistical tests.

Box 6.6 Dealing with borderline *p*-values, i.e. just above 0.05[13]

- Is the effect size clinically meaningful, and what benefits does it represent?
- Does most of the 95%CI lie in the region of benefit, e.g. relative risk CI 0.50–1.03?
- Do other outcome measures support a beneficial treatment effect?
- Is it a unique trial that is never to be repeated? A trial that has taken a long time or been conducted in a rare disorder could have an effect size that is clinically worthwhile.
- What are the consequences (harms) if the new intervention is used in practice but is truly ineffective?

Regression methods are powerful and efficient types of analyses. They can be used to:
- adjust for imbalances in baseline characteristics or other potential confounders
- adjust for the stratification factors used in randomising participants
- investigate an interaction between a treatment and a prognostic factor (subgroup analyses), or between two treatments (factorial trial)
- allow for repeated measures (the endpoint is measured several times on each person)
- handle missing data by using imputation.

Adjusting for baseline factors (covariates) can increase statistical power when the factors are moderately/strongly related to prognosis.

In addition to linear, logistic and Cox regressions, there are **Poisson regression** (endpoint is a count, e.g. number of hospital admissions per patient, or number of asthmatic attacks per patient), and **ordinal logistic regression** (endpoint is categorical with a natural ordering, e.g. disease severity is none, mild, moderate or severe).

There are also methods for **competing risks** (time-to-event outcomes).[18, 19] This is when participants have an event that prevents them from having the event of interest. For example, the primary trial endpoint could be death from cancer, but if someone dies from cardiovascular disease first they are not at risk of dying from cancer anymore. Cardiovascular disease is a competing risk. Standard time-to-event methods would consider the cardiovascular death the same as someone who is alive, i.e. both are censored. A common approach to deal with this issue is called the **cumulative incidence function**, which estimates the marginal probability (risk) of each type of event separately without censoring the cardiovascular deaths. It produces a hazard ratio for the effect of the new treatment on cancer, allowing for cardiovascular deaths occurring first; which is interpreted like any other hazard ratio.

Many statistical methods are referred to as **frequentist** (there is a *single* true but unknown value of the treatment effect, to be estimated by a trial). Other methods are **Bayesian statistics/methods**, which provide a distribution of probabilities over a *range* of plausible treatment effects, and they often incorporate prior evidence. They have been successfully used in several clinical trials, but are not commonly used because of their complexity, the difficulty in determining how much importance should be given to the previous evidence and quantifying it, and whether that evidence is reliable/applicable.

6.2 Safety, toxicity and adverse events

The efficacy benefits of any new intervention must be balanced against the safety profile, and this is most reliably done using a randomised trial.[20]

Analysing and reporting adverse events can be done in several ways.[21] One approach is to use all participants randomised (intention-to-treat analysis, see Section 6.5). But it could also be argued that the safety profile of a new treatment should only be based on those who took it (safety analysis dataset), because a *treatment-related* adverse event (i.e. one that is caused by the intervention) cannot occur in someone who did not take it. Both approaches could be used for a trial.

It should also be made clear whether the number of events (one person can be counted several times if they have multiple events of the same type) or number of people with an event (one person counted only once for an event type) is reported.

Table 6.3 is an example of selected adverse events and effect sizes for a clinical trial, noting that they occurred over an average of 41 months follow up.[22] It is important to

Table 6.3 The number of patients with specified adverse events from a randomised trial of bempedoic acid versus placebo for patients with cardiovascular disease who are statin intolerant. Source: Adapted from Nissen *et al.*[22]

	Bempedoic acid N = 7001 % (n)	Placebo N = 6964 % (n)	Relative risk	Absolute risk difference per 100	Number needed to harm (NNH)	P-value
Any adverse event	86.3 (6040)	85.0 (5919)	1.02	1.3 more	77	0.03
Any serious adverse event	25.2 (1767)	24.9 (1733)	1.01	0.3 more	333	0.63
Myalgia	5.6 (393)	6.8 (471)	0.82	1.2 fewer	83*	0.005
Gout	3.1 (215)	2.1 (143)	1.48	1.0 more	100	<0.0001
Hyperuricemia	10.9 (763)	5.6 (393)	1.92	5.3 more	19	<0.0001

* Treat 83 with bempedoic acid and there is 1 <u>less</u> case of myalgia.
Hyperuricemia: abnormally high uric acid in the blood.

Box 6.7 Analysing and interpreting adverse events

- Consider the impact of the events on participants: severity, whether easy or difficult to prevent (by prophylactic approaches) or treat, whether they negatively impact quality of life, and whether they lead to early stopping of the trial treatment or standard of care therapy (the latter could be an issue).
- Consider the costs of preventing or treating adverse events.
- Analyse all severity grades and/or the most severe grades.
- Analyse all reported events and also those *considered* related to (caused by) the treatment given. Giving only the latter could under-report adverse events, especially in unblinded trials where investigators may be biased in favour of the new treatment so less likely to assign a causal link for some events in this trial arm.
- Distinguish adverse events that are defined by biochemical measurements (e.g. liver or renal function, which might be asymptomatic) from those that have clinical symptoms (e.g. diarrhoea).
- Perhaps avoid giving p-values for every type of adverse event because of multiple testing (i.e. finding spurious statistically significant differences).

---

always look at the overall (total) adverse event rate (top row of Table 6.3), and then specific types. Box 6.7 provides general comments on analysing adverse events.

Number needed to harm (NNH) is calculated in the same way as number needed to treat (NNT, page 83), with the same limitations. It indicates the number of people given the new treatment to yield one extra (more) adverse event compared to controls (unless the new treatment is less harmful, e.g. myalgia Table 6.3). In very large trials, small clinical differences could be statistically significant (e.g. 'any adverse event' in Table 6.3) and so *p*-values need to be considered carefully.

Absolute risk differences provide a direct measure of impact so might be preferable to relative risks (or odds or hazards ratios) which can exaggerate the harm (e.g. hyperuricemia).

Some trial interventions have different exposure times which can influence the likelihood of adverse events (e.g. a new oral drug taken continuously for 12 months versus the control therapy which is a monthly injection of another drug for only 6 months). Similarly, for treatments taken continuously over time, the chance of experiencing an adverse event

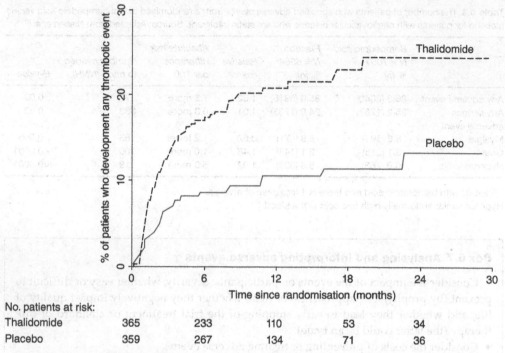

Figure 6.9 Example of a clinical trial of thalidomide versus placebo for patients with small-cell lung cancer on standard chemotherapy, where any thrombotic event was a major adverse event. Hazard ratio 2.13 (95%CI 1.41–2.30, $p < 0.001$.[24] Figure provided by the trial investigators (personal communication).

No. patients at risk:					
Thalidomide	365	233	110	53	34
Placebo	359	267	134	71	36

might increase with longer administration/exposure. Instead of using the number of participants as the denominator for risk, we can use number of person-years (see Section 'Incidence rate ratio', page 85). For example, in another trial of bempedoic acid versus placebo, patients could be taking daily drug for anywhere between 12 and 52 weeks (i.e. quite different exposure times).[23] The 2424 patients randomised to bemepdoic acid had 2026 total person-years, and the 1197 patients who had placebo had 1050 person-years. The number of patients who developed gout during the trial was 33 (bempedoic acid) and 5 (placebo). These become incidence rates of 1.6 per 100 person-years (33 out of 2026) and 0.5 per 100 person-years (5 out of 1050) respectively. The incidence rate ratio is then 3.20 (1.6 ÷ 0.5), and incidence rate difference is 1.1 extra case of gout per 100 person-years (1.6 − 0.5).

Occasionally the time it takes for an adverse event to occur is of interest. Fast onset of serious side effects could be a major issue. Kapan-Meier curves could be used to examine this. Figure 6.9 is an example where the effect on pulmonary embolism and deep vein thrombosis was seen quite soon after starting trial drug (thalidomide).[24]

6.3 Adherence (compliance)

For some interventions, adherence is easy to describe, such as when it is a one-off procedure, for example a new surgical technique (the person either had it or not). For others, adherence can require a more detailed definition, usually when the intervention is delivered as several sessions or continuously over time. Box 6.8 shows some considerations when interpreting adherence.

Box 6.8 Interpreting adherence

• How many participants stopped their allocated intervention early? Does this differ between the trial arms, and can this be explained?

• Summarise the main reasons why people stopped early in each group. Does any reason stand out, e.g. toxicity, unable to swallow the size of tablet/capsule, personal or clinician choice?

• How many participants had the dose (amount) of their allocated therapies reduced, delayed, interrupted or suspended (and what were the reasons)? Do these differ between the trial arms?

• Was adherence to standard concurrent therapies adversely affected?

Adherence can be analysed and presented in several ways. We can look at the mean (or median) time on a therapy, which is especially useful for drugs taken continuously (and daily). Kaplan-Meier curves can show this easily, where an 'event' is someone who stopped the trial therapy, and those who are still on it are censored at the date of last follow up. From the same trial shown in Figure 6.9, the median time on thalidomide or placebo was 6.8 or 7.9 months respectively.[24] Generally, if participants are on the new treatment longer than the control, this could reflect better efficacy and/or fewer side effects.

Adherence could be defined as someone who took the therapy for a certain proportion of time (e.g. they were meant to be on therapy for 12 months but only took it for 9 months, hence adherence is 75%). We could also use the percentage of the intended dose (e.g. person was meant to get 10 mg based on their body weight, but only received 6 mg for some reason, so they had 60% of the intended dose). If the trial therapies are given over a fixed schedule (e.g. month 0, 3 and 6) adherence can be easily displayed as the proportion of participants who received the treatment at each time point.

6.4 Health-related quality of life (QoL)

When evaluating efficacy outcomes, a goal of superiority trials is to show improvement (benefit) above that of the control therapy. Improving QoL is also an ideal goal, but in several cases (e.g. patients with advanced disease who are expected to deteriorate) even having a *stable* QoL is probably a positive finding. Indeed, this might be a goal when evaluating two drugs in combination compared to one drug, given the expected extra toxicities.

QoL instruments contain several questions. Each question often requires the participant to select one appropriate category, which has a numerical value. For example, in the Short Form-12 (SF-12) questionnaire one question is *During the past four weeks, how much of the time have you had any of the following problems with your work or other regular daily activities as a result of your physical health?* and the person has to select one of the following:

All of the time	Most of the time	Some of the time	A little of the time	None of the time
1	2	3	4	5

A total score for each participant can be obtained by simply summing the individual scores across all questions. Alternatively, the score for a group of questions is summed separately,

---

Box 6.9 Different ways of analysing QoL

1. Using its original value ('taking measurements on people').
2. Converted to time-to-event endpoints: time to QoL deterioration or improvement by a certain amount.
3. Converted to 'counting people' (binary) endpoints: percentage of people whose QoL deteriorates or improves.

They can sometimes produce what appears to be conflicting results. However, this is because they reflect different aspects of how a new therapy impacts QoL. The last two might be easier to explain, because it can be difficult to describe what an improvement in QoL score of e.g. 10 units 'feels' like. Choosing one or more approach depends on the research question being asked.

---

to produce a value for one of several domains. For example, the 12 questions on the SF-12 reduces to 8 domains[#], which can be reduced further to 2 ('physical' and 'mental').

The score for each participant is often transformed onto a continuous scale (e.g. ranges from 0 to 100). Detailed instructions on how to deal with raw scores and transform them are usually provided with the instrument.

QoL scores can be analysed in several ways including (Box 6.9)[25]:

1. *Using QoL as measured*

   Focus is on the change in QoL from baseline. There are statistical methods that allow a single analysis of all of the person's QoL values from all time points and for all participants (**repeated measures analysis** or **mixed modelling**). Figure 6.10 shows two examples of analysing QoL as a continuous measure: one shows the mean values at each time point and the other shows the scores averaged over time.[26, 27] Three pieces of information are required to interpret a treatment effect on QoL (Figure 6.10). The scale range is important. A mean difference between the new and control therapies of 5 units is big if the scale range is 0–20 but very small if on a scale range 0–150.

2. *Converting QoL to time-to-event*

   In Figure 6.11 QoL has been converted to a time-to-event endpoint.[28] Investigators pre-define what an event is, e.g. how much does the QoL score have to change from baseline for the person to be classified as having QoL deterioration (improvement in QoL can also be examined)? Hazard ratio and median times are interpreted in the same way as for efficacy (Section 'Outcome measures based on time-to-event data'). This approach can reflect fast deterioration/improvement, and some limitations are (using the example):

   • A decrease of 6 or 4 units probably have similar symptoms, but they would be classified respectively as an 'event' or 'no event'.
   • Someone whose score decreases by 6 units is considered the same as a decrease of 15.
   • Changing the cut-off to define an event could change the results.

3. *Converting QoL to 'counting people' endpoints*

   In the trial of lymphoma patients (and the FACT-Lymphoma subscale),[28] 86 among 139 patients (62%) given ibrutinib had a score that increased (improved) by ≥5 units, versus 50 among 141 control patients (35%). The relative risk for improving is 1.77 (62÷35) or absolute risk difference of 27 percentage points (62 – 35).

[#] General health, physical functioning, role physical, body pain, vitality, social functioning, role emotional, and mental health.

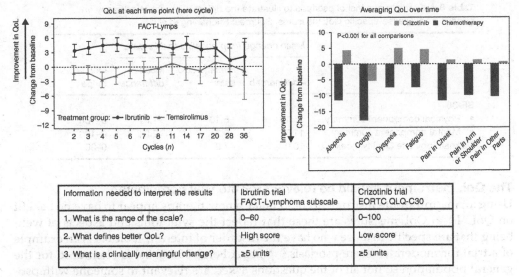

Information needed to interpret the results	Ibrutinib trial FACT-Lymphoma subscale	Crizotinib trial EORTC QLQ-C30
1. What is the range of the scale?	0–60	0–100
2. What defines better QoL?	High score	Low score
3. What is a clinically meaningful change?	≥5 units	≥5 units

Figure 6.10 Two trials that analyse QoL as a continuous measure: patients with relapsed or refractory mantle-cell lymphoma (left side; mean change and 95%CI at each time point) and patients with advanced non-small cell lung cancer that is ALK positive (right side; mean change averaged over time).[26, 27] The 'new' therapies are ibrutinib and crizotinib respectively. In both examples, the difference in QoL between the treatment arms reflect moderate effects that are clinically meaningful when considering the scale range and the minimum clinically important change. Figures reproduced with permission from Taylor & Francis/Leukemia and Lymphoma and the Massachusetts Medical Society/NEJM.

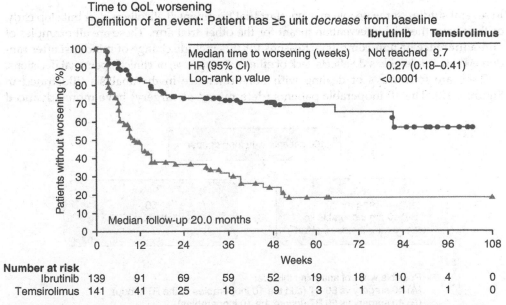

Figure 6.11 QoL (FACT Lymphoma subscale) is converted to a time-to-event endpoint, for the trial shown in Figure 6.10 (mantle-cell lymphoma). Source: Dreyling et al.[28] / figure reproduced with permission from Elsevier/Lancet. Patients who do not have the defined event (QoL worsens) could be censored at their last QoL assessment or clinic visit. HR = 0.27 means that the risk (hazard) of QoL getting worse with ibrutinib is lower than the controls, hence HR < 1.0 indicates benefit. If using time to QoL improvement instead, HR > 1.0 indicates benefit.

Table 6.4 Example of a trial of psoriasis to illustrate the different impact of a therapy on generic and disease-specific QoL measures. Sources: Sticherling et al.[29,30]

	Mean change from baseline to 24 weeks			
	Secukinumab	Fumaric acid ester	Mean difference	QoL score range
SF-36				
• Physical component summary	6.13	5.13	1.01	0–100
• Mental component summary	11.56	9.31	2.24	0–100
Dermatology Life Quality Index	−15.0	−7.9	−7.1	0–30

The QoL instrument should be relevant for the trial participants

Using an inappropriate instrument could make a new therapy appear to have no benefit on QoL. Ideal QoL measures are those that reflect the symptoms and aspects of well-being that are specific to those who have the disorder of interest. Table 6.4 is an example of a trial for moderate-severe psoriasis.[29, 30] Short Form-36 (SF-36) is often used for the general population so not all of the questions asked are relevant to someone with psoriasis; hence the lack of an effect of secukinumab on the two SF-36 domains. However, the Dermatology Life Quality Index (DLQI) is specifically for people suffering from skin diseases, covering items such as embarrassment, shopping and home care, and close relationships, and the impact of secukinumab was clear and large (mean difference of 7.1 on a scale 0–30).

6.5 Intention-to-treat and per-protocol analyses

In several studies, some people may not start trial treatment at all, others start but stop early, or they have the trial intervention meant for the other trial arm. These are all examples of **non-adherence** or **non-compliers**. Reasons for this include change of mind just after randomisation, intolerable side-effects, lack of efficacy/ response, or clinical/personal decisions.

There are four ways of dealing with non-adherence in the analysis (illustrated in Figure 6.12). The 10 inoperable patients (determined at surgery) have more advanced

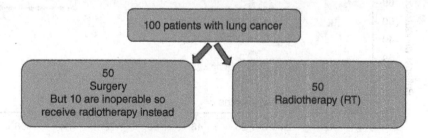

Possible ways of analysing this are:
(A) 40 surgery vs 60 RT (add the 10 inoperables to the RT group)
(B) 40 surgery vs 50 RT (ignore the 10 inoperables)
(C) 40 surgery vs 40 RT (remove equivalent 10 from the RT group)
(D) 50 surgery vs 50 RT (leave the 10 inoperables in the surgery group)

Figure 6.12 Hypothetical trial comparing two treatments in 100 patients with lung cancer, illustrating possible ways to deal with non-adherence to the allocated treatment. The main outcome is survival at 1 year.

disease, and therefore poorer survival. Options A and B involve moving people around or ignoring these 'worst' patients, making surgery seem better than it really is. In Option C, it is difficult to identify and remove 10 *equivalent* patients in the radiotherapy group to the 10 inoperable patients in the surgery group. Options A to C disrupt the balance achieved by randomisation, thus creating bias. Only option D maintains balanced baseline characteristics – called **intention-to-treat analysis (ITT)**. Participants are analysed according to the group to which they were randomised, regardless of whether they took the allocated intervention or not, but this can produce a diluted treatment effect. The effect size might reflect non-adherence as seen in routine practice. The scientific advantage of having two balanced trial arms, with minimal bias, outweighs a potentially underestimated effect size. All trials should be analysed using ITT.

A **per-protocol analysis** only includes participants who took their allocated treatment as specified in the trial protocol (Option B in Figure 6.12); acknowledging that some balance in participants' characteristics may be lost. Different definitions of adherence (Section 6.3, page 98) could be applied to see whether treatment effects are similar or better in subgroups of participants with 'good/high' adherence compared to that in all participants.

6.6 Summary points

- A summary effect size can be obtained for any comparison of two interventions.
- The type of effect size and how it is analysed depends on the type of outcome measure – counting people, taking measurements or time-to-event data:
  - Counting people: absolute risk difference, relative risk, odds ratio
  - Taking measurements on people: difference between two means or medians
  - Time-to-event: hazard ratio, difference between two survival or event rates (proportions).
- Confidence intervals and p-values for any effect size help to fully interpret the data.
- Efficacy, adverse events, adherence and health-related quality of life are key outcomes to be analysed. The benefit-harm balance (particularly between efficacy and adverse events) need to be considered and agreed between the investigators before recommending a new intervention.
- Clear positive effects for primary endpoints are strengthened further by beneficial effects on secondary endpoints.
- All trials should be analysed using intention-to-treat, unless otherwise justified.

References

1. Petrie A, Sabine C. *Medical Statistics at a Glance*. 4th edn, Wiley-Blackwell, 2019.
2. Kirkwood B, Sterne J. *Essential Medical Statistics*. 3rd edn, Wiley-Blackwell, 2019.
3. Govaert TME, Thijs CTMCN, Masurel N et al. The efficacy of influenza vaccination in elderly individuals. *JAMA* 1994; **272**(21): 1661–1665.
4. Saver JL, Lewis RJ. Number needed to treat: conveying the likelihood of a therapeutic effect. *JAMA*. 2019; **321**(8):798–799.
5. Gardner CD, Trepanowski JF, Del Gobbo LC, Hauser ME, Rigdon J, Ioannidis JPA, Desai M, King AC. Effect of low-fat vs low-carbohydrate diet on 12-month weight loss in overweight adults and the association with genotype pattern or insulin secretion: the DIETFITS randomized clinical trial. *JAMA*. 2018; **319**(7):667–679.

6. Vickers AJ, Altman DG. Analysing controlled trials with baseline and follow-up measurements. *BMJ* 2001; **323**:1123–1124.

7. Guideline on adjustment for baseline covariates in clinical trials. European Medicines Agency. EMA/CHMP/295050/2013.

8. Insogna KL, Briot K, Imel EA *et al.*; AXLES 1 Investigators. A randomized, double-blind, placebo-controlled, phase 3 trial evaluating the efficacy of burosumab, an anti-FGF23 antibody, in adults with X-linked hypophosphatemia: week 24 primary analysis. *J Bone Miner Res.* 2018; **33**(8):1383–1393.

9. Powles T, Park SH, Voog E *et al.* Avelumab maintenance therapy for advanced or metastatic urothelial carcinoma. *N Engl J Med.* 2020; **383**(13):1218–1230.

10. Moore MJ, Goldstein D, Hamm J *et al.*; National Cancer Institute of Canada Clinical Trials Group. Erlotinib plus gemcitabine compared with gemcitabine alone in patients with advanced pancreatic cancer: a phase III trial of the National Cancer Institute of Canada Clinical Trials Group. *J Clin Oncol.* 2007; **25**(15):1960–1966.

11. Sabatine MS, Giugliano RP, Keech AC *et al.*; FOURIER Steering Committee and Investigators. Evolocumab and clinical outcomes in patients with cardiovascular disease. *N Engl J Med.* 2017; **376**(18):1713–1722.

12. Dehbi HM, Royston P, Hackshaw A. Life expectancy difference and life expectancy ratio: two measures of treatment effects in randomised trials with non-proportional hazards. *BMJ* 2017; **357**:j2250.

13. Hackshaw A, Kirkwood A. Research and methods: interpreting and reporting clinical trials with results of borderline statistical significance. *BMJ* 2011; **343**. doi: https://doi.org/10.1136/bmj.d3340.

14. Greenland S, Senn SJ, Rothman KJ, Carlin JB, Poole C, Goodman SN, Altman DG. Statistical tests, P values, confidence intervals, and power: a guide to misinterpretations. *Eur J Epidemiol.* 2016; **31**(4):337–350.

15. The ASA's statement on p-values: context, process and purpose (American Statistical Association). The American Statistician 2016; **70**(2): 219–233.

16. Greenland S. Valid p-values behave exactly as they should: some misleading criticisms of p-values and their resolution with S-values. *The American Statistician* 2019; **73**(51): 106–114.

17. Wasserstein RL, Schirm AL, Lazar NA. Moving to a world beyond "p<0.05". *The American Statistician* 2019; **73** (S1): 1–29.

18. Austin PC, Lee DS, Fine JP. Introduction to the analysis of survival data in the presence of competing risks. *Circulation.* 2016; **133**(6):601–609.

19. Huebner M, Wolkewitz M, Enriquez-Sarano M *et al.* Competing risks need to be considered in survival analysis models for cardiovascular outcomes. *J Thorac Cardiovasc Surg.* 2017; **153**(6):1427–1431.

20. Collins R, MacMahon S. Reliable assessment of the effects of treatment on mortality and major morbidity, I: clinical trials. *The Lancet* 2001; **357**: 373–380.

21 Lineberry N, Berlin JA, Mansi B, Glasser S. Recommendations to improve adverse event reporting in clinical trial publications: a joint pharmaceutical industry/journal editor perspective. *BMJ* 2016; 355. doi: https://doi.org/10.1136/bmj.i5078.

22. Nissen SE, Lincoff AM, Brennan D *et al.*; CLEAR Outcomes Investigators. Bempedoic acid and cardiovascular outcomes in statin-intolerant patients. *N Engl J Med.* 2023; **388**(15):1353–1364.

23. Bays HE, Banach M, Catapano AL *et al.* Bempedoic acid safety analysis: pooled data from four phase 3 clinical trials. *J Clin Lipidol.* 2020; **14**(5):649–659.

24. Lee SM, Woll PJ, Rudd R *et al.* Anti-angiogenic therapy using thalidomide combined with chemotherapy in small cell lung cancer: a randomized, double-blind, placebo-controlled trial. *J Natl Cancer Inst* 2009; **101**(15):1049–1057.

25. Fayers PM, Machin D. *Quality of Life: The Assessment, Analysis and Reporting of Patient-reported Outcomes.* 3rd edn, Wiley-Blackwell, 2015

26. Hess G, Rule S, Jurczak W *et al.* Health-related quality of life data from a phase 3, international, randomized, open-label, multicenter study in patients with previously treated mantle cell lymphoma treated with ibrutinib versus temsirolimus. *Leuk Lymphoma.* 2017; **58**(12):2824–2832.

27. Shaw AT, Kim DW, Nakagawa K *et al.* Crizotinib versus chemotherapy in advanced ALK-positive lung cancer. *N Engl J Med.* 2013; **368**(25):2385–2394.

28. Dreyling M, Jurczak W, Jerkeman M *et al*. Ibrutinib versus temsirolimus in patients with relapsed or refractory mantle-cell lymphoma: an international, randomised, open-label, phase 3 study. *Lancet.* 2016; **387**(10020):770–778.

29. Sticherling M, Mrowietz U, Augustin M *et al*. Secukinumab is superior to fumaric acid esters in treating patients with moderate-to-severe plaque psoriasis who are naive to systemic treatments: results from the randomized controlled PRIME trial. *Br J Dermatol.* 2017; **177**(4):1024–1032.

30. Institute for Quality and Efficiency in Health Care (IQWiG). Dossier assessment of Secukinumab (Plaque-Psoriasis) (A17-08). `https://www.iqwig.de/download/a17-08_secukinumab_ extract-of-dossier-assessment_v1-0.pdf`.

CHAPTER 7

Randomised trials – additional aspects of analysis and interpretation

This chapter builds on Chapter 6 by outlining additional specific topics that may not apply to all trials, covering:

- Non-inferiority studies
- Composite outcome measures
- Subgroup analyses
- Crossover, factorial and cluster randomised trials
- Repeated measurements of the outcome measure
- Multiple endpoints
- Missing data
- Analysing biomarkers (translational research).

Textbooks[1,2] and the reading list (page 205) provide more information and discussion.

7.1 Non-inferiority and equivalence trials

Showing superiority of one treatment over another is relatively easy; Box 7.1. However, the interpretation of equivalence and non-inferiority trials is driven by the maximum allowable difference or non-inferiority margin (see Chapter 6) and where the observed confidence interval (CI) (i.e. the *true* treatment effect) lies in relation to this pre-specified margin (Box 7.1). These trial types need to be large enough to produce precise estimates of treatment effect, to yield narrow CIs.

The example in Box 7.2 and Figure 7.1 shows how to interpret equivalence or non-inferiority studies using CIs. Because confidence intervals indicate what the *true effect* might be, the whole CI range needs to be below the pre-specified margin in order to conclude non-inferiority. In that trial,[3] the non-inferiority margin was +5 units; therefore, any difference above this indicates that the average Yale-Brown score among people given telephone therapy would be unacceptably high (a high score indicates worse symptoms).

Figure 7.1 shows how conclusions can vary depending on where the CI lies in relation to the non-inferiority (allowable) margin. In the trial, the observed upper 95%CI limit is +4.26, suggesting that the true effect of telephone therapy could be a bit worse than face-to-face therapy. However, this loss of efficacy is within the margin of +5 units and so is considered worthwhile given the benefit (easier access to therapy). Telephone

A Concise Guide to Clinical Trials, Second Edition. Allan Hackshaw.
© 2024 John Wiley & Sons Ltd. Published 2024 by John Wiley & Sons Ltd.

Box 7.1 Interpreting trials comparing interventions A and B

Objective	Objective is met when
Superiority (A is more effective than B)	95% confidence interval excludes the no-effect value and p-value < 0.05.
Equivalence (A has a similar effect to B)	Confidence interval includes the no-effect value and the interval is completely within the allowable difference
Non-inferiority (A has an effect not much worse than B)	Confidence interval does not cross one end of the allowable difference (i.e. the end that indicates 'A' is worse)

Box 7.2 Example of a phase III non-inferiority trial comparing two methods of delivering cognitive behavioural therapy to people with obsessive-compulsive disorder (OCD). Source: Lovell et al.[3]

Location: 2 psychology outpatient departments in the UK

Participants: 72 individuals aged ≥16 years with obsessive-compulsive disorder

Intervention: Cognitive behaviour therapy (10 weekly sessions) delivered by telephone.

Control: Cognitive behaviour therapy (10 weekly sessions) delivered face-to-face in the clinic

Outcome measure: Yale-Brown obsessive compulsive score (range 0–40, high score indicates more severe symptoms)

Justification for trial: 'Face-to-face' therapy involves waiting lists and some people are unable to attend clinic appointments. Delivering therapy by telephone should increase access to treatment

Trial objective: 'Telephone' is non-inferior to 'face-to-face' therapy

Non-inferiority margin: mean difference +5 units (Yale-Brown score)

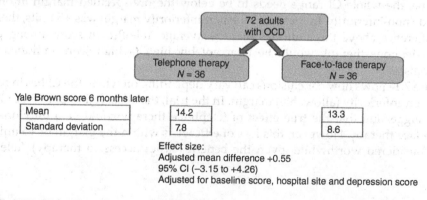

- The 95% CI for the *true* mean difference is between −3.15 and +4.26 units
- This is below +5 units, so 'telephone' is considered **not inferior**
- However, the 95% CI is completely within the noninferiority margin of ±5 units, so it can also be concluded that the two interventions have an **equivalent** effect.

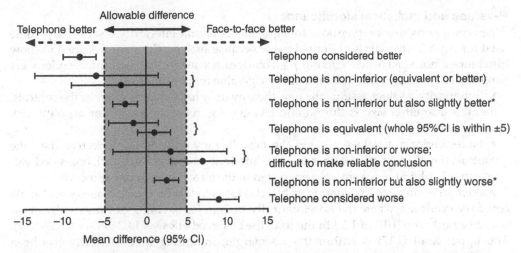

Figure 7.1 Illustration of interpreting effect sizes and confidence intervals from equivalence or non-inferiority trials using the example in Box 7.2, where the maximum allowable difference (non-inferiority margin) is five units shown by the shading. Mean difference = mean score using 'telephone' minus mean score using 'face-to-face' delivery. *Although statistically significant it might not be clinically important because the effect and whole 95%CI are within ±5 units.

therapy can be recommended. If the lower CI limit had exceeded +5 units we would conclude that the possible true effect is unacceptable, and telephone therapy would not be recommended.

Intention-to-treat (ITT) and per-protocol analyses

ITT is the standard analysis for superiority trials. However, for equivalence or non-inferiority trials, the inclusion of people who did not have the randomised intervention could bias the results; Table 7.1. Therefore, a per-protocol analysis is often used in addition to an ITT analysis, but in some non-inferiority and equivalence trials it is the primary analysis.

Table 7.1 Illustration of how intention-to-treat (ITT) analyses can 'bias' results towards a non-inferiority conclusion. Assume non-adherers (i.e. who did not take the randomised therapy) had similar characteristics and the same standard of care and outcomes as the controls (outside of the trial).

| | Outcome is death rate % (number) | | | Allowable margin is +10% |
	New therapy	Control	Risk difference	Conclusion
Adherers (**per protocol**):	33% (200/600)	20% (120/600)	+13%	New therapy is inferior (worse) than control
Non-adherers	25% (100/400)	25% (100/400)	0	
Everyone (**ITT**):	30% (300/1000)	22% (220/1000)	+8%	New therapy is non-inferior to control

P-values and statistical significance

When comparing two interventions for equivalence or non-inferiority, a standard p-value used for superiority trials is of limited value because such p-values are designed to show differences, not similarities. Having $p \geq 0.05$ does *not* mean that two interventions are similarly effective. Instead, there is a specific p-value for non-inferiority.

- Superiority p-values assume the new therapy truly has the same effect as the controls, (i.e. the true effect size is the no effect value, e.g. relative risk 1.0, or absolute risk difference 0).
- Non-inferiority p-values assume the new therapy truly is less effective than the controls (i.e. the true effect size is the non-inferiority margin or greater); one-sided values are used because we are only interested in the effect being in one direction.

Consider an example of lixisenatide vs placebo for people with type 2 diabetes and acute coronary syndrome where the non-inferiority margin for having a cardiovascular event was a hazard ratio (HR) of 1.3.[4] In the trial, the observed HR was 1.02 (95% CI 0.89-1.17). The upper limit (1.17) is within the 1.3 margin, indicating non-inferiority has been met. The non-inferiority p-value is <0.001. Assuming the true HR is ≥ 1.3, the likelihood of seeing a HR of 1.02 or lower due to chance is less than 1 in 1000 trials of a similar size and design. Because this is unlikely to occur we conclude non-inferiority and the treatment could be recommended. Had we instead observed a HR of 1.18 with non-inferiority p-value=0.15, the likelihood of seeing a HR of 1.18 or lower by chance is 15 in 100 similar trials, hence this HR is consistent with the margin of 1.3, so non-inferiority could *not* be concluded and the treatment not recommended.

Can we switch between non-inferiority and superiority?

Because a non-inferiority trial is larger than a corresponding superiority trial, there should be enough statistical power to conclude either non-inferiority or superiority. In another trial of type 2 diabetes (canagliflozin vs placebo) the observed HR was 0.86 (95%CI 0.75-0.97).[5] The non-inferiority p-value was <0.001 (so this objective was met), but the superiority p-value was 0.02 (and the 95%CI excludes 1.0). Here, we can switch the conclusion from non-inferiority to superiority. The reverse cannot be done generally, because a superiority study is unlikely to be large enough to produce a narrow CI that excludes the non-inferiority margin; also the margin would often not have been pre-specified.

7.2 Composite outcome measures

Composite endpoints increase the number of events and therefore the likelihood of achieving $p < 0.05$. They also avoid issues over multiplicity when analysing each component separately. Although the main trial conclusion should be based on the pre-specified composite primary endpoint, investigators often show results for each component. Ideally, the new treatment has similar effects across the components, regardless of being statistically significant. Table 7.2 is an example where the treatment effect appears to differ.[6]

The overall effect was clear (HR 0.74). However, at first glance, semaglutide appears beneficial for non-fatal stroke (0.61) only, possibly effective for non-fatal myocardial infarction (0.74 but $p = 0.12$), and completely ineffective[#] for CVD deaths (0.98).

[#] 'Ineffective' as in semaglutide has the same effect as placebo.

Table 7.2 An example of interpreting a composite outcome measure (trial of treating type 2 diabetes). Source: Marso *et al.*[6]

	Semaglutide N = 1648	Placebo N = 1649		
	No. of events		Hazard ratio (95% CI)	P-value
Primary composite*	108	146	0.74 (0.58–0.95)	0.02
Components				
Death from CVD	44	46	0.98 (0.65–1.48)	0.92
Non-fatal myocardial infarction	47	64	0.74 (0.51–1.08)	0.12
Non-fatal stroke	27	44	0.61 (0.38–0.99)	0.04

CVD: cardiovascular disease.
* Death or non-fatal myocardial infarction or stroke.

But can we make claims only about the individual component that showed a statistically significant effect and ignore the others? The answer is often 'no'. The lack of an observed benefit or statistical significance could be due to a small number of events (and chance). Also, there may be no reliable biological rationale why the treatment is beneficial for only some components.

Although CVD death has a HR of 0.98, the 95%CI (what the true effect might be) is very wide. Importantly, it goes down to a lower limit of 0.65 (potential benefit) and the interval easily contains HR 0.74, which is consistent with the overall effect. If the Kaplan–Meier curves for CVD death completely overlapped, this might suggest no effect (compared to placebo), but the data still lack reliability and statistical power.

The trial investigators concluded that semaglutide was effective for reducing CVD, with the clarification that most of the effect *might* be driven by non-fatal stroke and to a lesser extent non-fatal myocardial infarction. It seemed reasonable to not make definitive claims.

7.3 Subgroup (subset) analyses

Investigators frequently undertake subgroup analyses, which involve examining the effect size in separate groups of participants usually defined by a baseline characteristic or bio- or imaging marker. Occasionally subgroup analyses are used as a 'fishing expedition' to find a positive/beneficial effect when the overall effect shows little/no difference. There are essentially four potential conclusions from subgroup analyses (Figure 7.2). The top outcome in Figure 7.2 is an acceptable use of subgroup analyses (i.e. no clear evidence that the treatment effect differs between the groups, which is what most of us aim for), while the second example (HR 0.75 versus 0.45) just provides additional information about the treatment.[#]

However, when subgroup analyses are used to determine who will and will not receive the new treatment (lower two outcomes of Figure 7.2), there needs to be convincing evidence to avoid withholding an effective therapy from future individuals. Subgroup factors can be pre-specified in the trial protocol or selected at the end of the trial (*post hoc*).

[#] These effects can be considered alongside treatment costs to possibly justify using the new treatment only in the subgroup with the biggest effect because it is the most cost-effective.

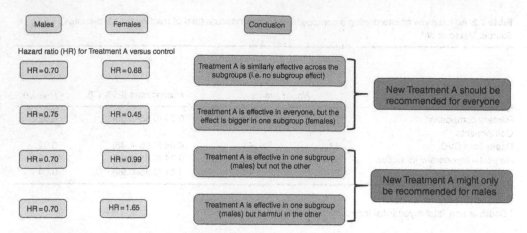

Figure 7.2 Four possible outcomes of subgroup analyses. HR (hazard ratio; but could also be relative risk or odds ratio) is for an outcome that is bad (e.g. death or disease event). RR<1 means that New Treatment A is more beneficial than the control. For the bottom two outcomes, the 95%CIs for females should ideally exclude a clinically meaningful benefit to be reliable (e.g. lower limit HR>0.95).

Although pre-specified factors are preferable, *post hoc* ones can be valid when justified using the scientific literature, and it is acceptable to examine the factors for hypothesis generation.

Subgroup analyses are presented as a **forest plot** (Figure 7.3).[7] A common approach is to see whether each treatment effect is statistically significant or not (i.e. whether the subgroup 95%CI overlaps the no-effect value or not). This could be done for sex in Figure 7.3, in which it appears that the drug T-DXd has a clear benefit among males but not in females. However, investigators mistakenly translate this as the treatment is effective in one subgroup and not the other. The observed overall effect size is the best estimate of the treatment effect, so this is what subgroups should be compared with, and we also make use of the definition of confidence intervals (what the **true effect size** is likely to be).

One simple (descriptive) approach is to see whether any subgroup 95%CI does not overlap the 95%CI for the overall effect size ('primary cohort'). In Figure 7.3, this would involve a shaded box covering HR 0.39–0.88, and seeing whether any subgroup 95%CI lies outside of this, which is not the case here. This strict approach makes it difficult to claim subgroup effects.

There are two fundamentally different statistical tests, where the questions are phrased to conclude 'no subgroup effect'[8, 9]:

- Is each subgroup effect size *consistent with the overall effect* (each 95%CI includes the overall effect size)?
- Are subgroup effect sizes not statistically significantly *different from each other* (test for interaction *p*-value is≥0.05, often using regression methods)?

Evidence for a subgroup effect is when one or more of the 95%CIs do not include the overall effect size *and* the test for interaction *p*-value<0.05, but ideally *p* < 0.001 to reflect strong evidence as multiple subgroup factors are often examined.

There is a general lack of clarity over using these two tests; either or both are reported. Figure 7.3 shows the vertical dashed line for the overall effect, but when this is missing it is easy to draw on by hand with a ruler. Box 7.3 shows the interpretation of subgroup analyses using three factors from the example in Figure 7.3.

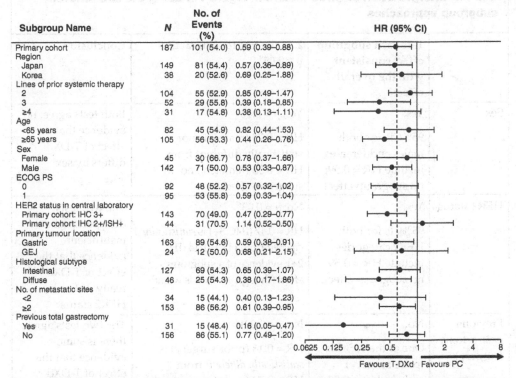

Subgroup Name	N	No. of Events (%)	HR (95% CI)
Primary cohort	187	101 (54.0)	0.59 (0.39–0.88)
Region			
Japan	149	81 (54.4)	0.57 (0.36–0.89)
Korea	38	20 (52.6)	0.69 (0.25–1.88)
Lines of prior systemic therapy			
2	104	55 (52.9)	0.85 (0.49–1.47)
3	52	29 (55.8)	0.39 (0.18–0.85)
≥4	31	17 (54.8)	0.38 (0.13–1.11)
Age			
<65 years	82	45 (54.9)	0.82 (0.44–1.53)
≥65 years	105	56 (53.3)	0.44 (0.26–0.76)
Sex			
Female	45	30 (66.7)	0.78 (0.37–1.66)
Male	142	71 (50.0)	0.53 (0.33–0.87)
ECOG PS			
0	92	48 (52.2)	0.57 (0.32–1.02)
1	95	53 (55.8)	0.59 (0.33–1.04)
HER2 status in central laboratory			
Primary cohort: IHC 3+	143	70 (49.0)	0.47 (0.29–0.77)
Primary cohort: IHC 2+/ISH+	44	31 (70.5)	1.14 (0.52–0.50)
Primary tumour location			
Gastric	163	89 (54.6)	0.59 (0.38–0.91)
GEJ	24	12 (50.0)	0.68 (0.21–2.15)
Histological subtype			
Intestinal	127	69 (54.3)	0.65 (0.39–1.07)
Diffuse	46	25 (54.3)	0.38 (0.17–1.86)
No. of metastatic sites			
<2	34	15 (44.1)	0.40 (0.13–1.23)
≥2	153	86 (56.2)	0.61 (0.39–0.95)
Previous total gastrectomy			
Yes	31	15 (48.4)	0.16 (0.05–0.47)
No	156	86 (55.1)	0.77 (0.49–1.20)

0.0625   0.125   0.25   0.5   1   2   4   8
Favours T-DXd   Favours PC

Figure 7.3 Forest plot showing subgroup analyses in a randomised trial of patients with advanced HER-2 positive gastric cancer comparing trastuzumab deruxtecan (T-DXd) with physician's choice (PC) chemotherapy. Effect size is hazard ratio (HR) for overall survival. The vertical dashed line is the hazard ratio among everyone (0.59). ECOG PS, Eastern Cooperative Oncology Group performance status; GEJ, gastroesophageal junction; HER2, human epidermal growth factor receptor 2; IHC, immunohistochemistry; ISH, in situ hybridisation. Source: Shitara et al.[7]/figure reproduced with permission from the Massachusetts Medical Society/NEJM.

If the effect size point estimate is close to the no effect value, even with a wide 95%CI, the harm-benefit balance and costs could be considered with a conservative recommendation to not use the new therapy for that particular subgroup, especially if there are side effects.

Box 7.4 outlines the statistical and non-statistical evidence that should be considered if there are real and reliable subgroup effects. Another vital piece of information is **biological plausibility**. In a trial of aspirin vs placebo among 17,000 patients with suspected acute myocardial infarction, the overall relative risk was 0.80 ($p<0.0001$).[10] The effect was 1.09 (95%CI 0.88-1.35) for people with a Libra/Gemini astrological star sign, and 0.74 (95%CI 0.68-0.82) for all other star signs. Both subgroup statistical tests were met (interaction p-value = 0.001, so 1.09 is statistically significantly different from 0.74; and the 95%CI for Libra/Gemini excludes the overall relative risk of 0.80). However, there is no biological plausibility for this subgroup effect whatsoever. The investigators deliberately performed numerous subgroup analyses to show that by doing so spurious effects can be found by chance.[#]

[#] With $p = 0.05$ (5%) we expect to find 1 in 20 subgroup analyses to produce spurious effects (by chance) when there really is no subgroup effect.

Box 7.3 Interpretation of three factors in Figure 7.3 using the two different subgroup approaches

	1. Is each subgroup effect consistent with the overall effect?	2. Is the test for interaction $p \geq 0.05^*$	Conclusion
Sex	Yes. 95%CIs for both males and females include HR = 0.59; no subgroup effect.	Yes; $p = 0.18^*$ HR = 0.78 (males) is not statistically different from HR = 0.53 (females); no subgroup effect	Both tests agree: no evidence that the effect of T-DXd differs by sex
HER2 status	Yes. 95%CIs for both HER2 categories include HR = 0.59; no subgroup effect.	No; $p = 0.03^*$ HR = 0.47 (IHC 3+) is *statistically different* from HR = 1.14 (IHC 2+); evidence of a subgroup effect (though $p = 0.03$ is weak)	The two tests disagree: probably insufficient evidence that the effect of T-DXd really differs by HER2 status
Previous gastrectomy (surgery)	No. One of the 95%CIs (prior surgery) *excludes* HR = 0.59; evidence of a subgroup effect.	No; $p < 0.001^*$ HR = 0.16 (prior surgery) is *statistically different* from HR = 0.77 (no prior surgery); evidence of a subgroup effect	The two tests agree: there is some evidence that the effect of T-DXd differs by prior surgery or not

*p-values were estimated from the results.

Box 7.4 Evidence for concluding that there is a genuine subgroup effect, i.e. the new treatment should/could only be given to some people and not others. Source: Adapted from Dehbi and Hackshaw[9]

- Both statistical tests (Box 7.3) should be met (statistical evidence), and the interaction p-value should ideally be <0.001.
- There should be biological plausibility.
- There should be independent (corroborating) evidence from other studies.

Other considerations are :
- With numerous subgroup factors multiplicity should be allowed for.*
- Dividing the data into small subgroups (few participants or few events) can produce unreliable results.
- Baseline characteristics may no longer be balanced for a subgroup factor (creating confounding).

*E.g. in Figure 7.3 there are 10 subgroup analyses. The interaction p-value for HER2 status is 0.03 (Box 7.3) so a Bonferroni correction for multiplicity means that $p = 0.03$ becomes $p = 0.30$ (0.03×10). Whereas the p-value for prior surgery is <0.001, which becomes <0.01 after adjustment which is still significant (hence why a very small interaction p-value is best).

7.4 Crossover trials

Here, all participants receive all the interventions. When the endpoint is 'taking measurements on people', each participant has two values (new intervention and control), and the difference can be taken, or a regression analysis could be used to adjust for the baseline value. The effect size is the mean of these differences over all participants. Interpretation is the same as a mean difference from a two-arm trial (see page 85), and a 95% CI and p-value are calculated.

If the trial endpoint is based on counting people, a 2×2 table can be constructed (Table 7.3). Patients who had an exacerbation on both interventions ($n = 8$) or had no exacerbations at all ($n = 74$) reveal nothing about whether treatment A is more effective than a placebo. However, the numbers representing discordant results are informative (6 vs 12); the **odds ratio** is 0.5 (6/12).[#] The odds of suffering an exacerbation on Treatment A is half that on placebo. Statistical methods are available to calculate a 95% CI and p-value for the odds ratio. Time-to-event endpoints are rarely, if ever, used in crossover trials.

The analysis of crossover trials can also allow for a **period effect**; i.e. whether the effect size for Treatment B when preceded by A is different from Treatment A when preceded by B. Furthermore, although the time interval between treatments should be long enough to minimise a **carryover effect** from one treatment to the next, there are statistical methods that can allow for this.

7.5 Factorial trials

A factorial trial can efficiently compare two or more new interventions. Table 7.4 shows the results from a trial evaluating folic acid and other multivitamins in preventing neural tube defect pregnancies.[11] A large (71%) risk reduction was associated with folic acid (relative risk 0.29), with a small p-value, but there was no evidence of an effect with other vitamins. The conclusion was to recommend folic acid only.

Factorial trials can also be used to detect an **interaction** between two interventions, i.e. the effect size for one treatment depends on whether the person has received the other treatment or not; Figure 7.4. Statistical (regression) methods can be used to investigate interactions, and provide p-values for them. Figure 7.5 is another example of a factorial trial (low event rates indicate benefit).[12] The four individual Kaplan–Meier curves and the two main comparisons are shown (apixaban and placebo each have the lowest event rates). Even though the vitamin K antagonist plus aspirin had the highest event rates (i.e. the most harmful), there was no interaction effect between the therapies ($p = 0.64$);

Table 7.3 Hypothetical results from a crossover trial comparing Treatment A with placebo in 100 patients with asthma. The outcome measure is the occurrence of an exacerbation or not.

		Placebo	
		Exacerbation	No exacerbation
Treatment A	Exacerbation	8	12
	No exacerbation	6	74

[#] This has a different calculation to the odds ratio from a two-arm trial (Table 7.3).

Table 7.4 Randomised double-blind factorial trial comparing folic acid and other multivitamins in preventing neural tube defect (NTD) pregnancies in 1195 women. Source: the MRC Vitamin Study [11]

Trial treatment		Number with an NTD pregnancy/ number in trial arm (%)	Relative risk (RR) calculation	
Folic acid	Other vitamins		Folic acid vs no folic acid	Other vitamins vs no other vitamins
Yes	No	2/298 (0.7)	$RR = \dfrac{(2+4)/(298+295)}{(13+8)/(300+302)}$	$RR = \dfrac{(4+8)/(295+302)}{(2+13)/(298+300)}$
Yes	Yes	4/295 (1.4)	= 0.29	= 0.80
No	No	13/300 (4.3)	95% CI = 0.12–0.71	95% CI = 0.38–1.70
No	Yes	8/302 (2.6)	p-value <0.0001	p-value = 0.70

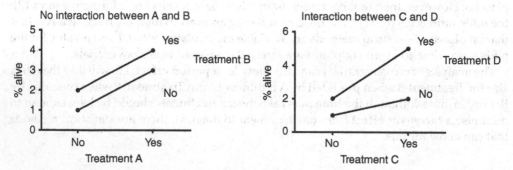

Figure 7.4 Illustration of an interaction between two treatments. In the left-hand figure, the effect of Treatment A does not depend on whether B was given or not (i.e. combining A and B has the same effect as adding (summing) the separate effects of A and B). But in the right-hand figure, the effect of Treatment C depends on whether D was given or not (i.e. combining C and D produces a greater effect than summing the separate effects of C and D).

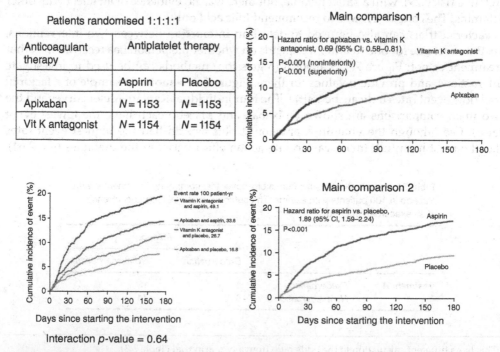

Figure 7.5 Example of a factorial trial in patients with atrial fibrillation (the primary outcome event is major or clinically relevant nonmajor bleeding). Source: Lopes et al.[12]/figure reproduced with permission from the Massachusetts Medical Society/NEJM.

i.e. the combined effect of vitamin K antagonist and aspirin is consistent with adding the effects when used on their own. When a clear interaction exists the effect size for *each* treatment combination should be reported.

7.6 Cluster randomised trial

The analyses described above apply to trials in which individual participants are randomised to the trial interventions. In a cluster randomised trial including stepped wedge designs, *groups* of people are randomised to each intervention (see page 66). A trial comparing two educational programmes could randomise schools to programme A or B. All children in the same school receive the same intervention. Variability exists between children in the same school, and between schools. Analysing the trial as if the children themselves were randomised assumes independence in their responses. However, children within a school may be more similar than children between schools. Allowance should be made for this within-school variability (the **intra-class correlation**).

Suppose all children in a particular school have the same test score. Assessing more than one child from each school adds no information, and the number of independent observations would equal the number of schools. However, in reality, there would be variability within a school. By ignoring the within-school (intra-class) correlation, the *p*-value for an effect size could be smaller than it should be, producing a statistically significant result and an incorrect conclusion.[13, 14] However, if the number of people within a cluster is small, the within-cluster variation may have a minimal effect, and the results of the trial could be similar to those obtained by assuming the data came from a standard trial where participants themselves were randomised.

7.7 Repeated measures

When several measurements of the same endpoint ('taking measurements on people', continuous data) are taken on each participant over time, they are likely to be correlated, and the effect size and *p*-value need to allow for this. A **repeated measures analysis of variance** or **covariance** can be performed. The analysis could produce a single *p*-value for comparing the two interventions and *p*-values for each time point, which accounts for multiple comparisons. **Mixed modelling** is a sophisticated statistical method used for this type of data with a similar underlying principle as linear regression. These methods produce a mean difference, interpreted in the same way as when only one measurement per person exists.

A similar concept can be used when the outcome is 'counting people', but the event can occur several times for a person, for example an infection. Methods for logistic regression can be used (generalised estimating equations), which produce odds ratios.

7.8 Multiple endpoints

Some trials have several major endpoints (or a single primary outcome and multiple key secondary endpoints). The more comparisons performed on the same data, the more likely that a spurious effect is found, i.e. an effect size with a *p*-value <0.05, but the effect was due to chance. When there are multiple primary outcome measures, any *p*-value <0.05 could be adjusted using simple methods such as a **Bonferroni correction**.[15, 16] A *p*-value of 0.02 becomes 0.06 if there are three comparisons (0.02×3). However, this assumes the outcome measures are uncorrelated, which may not be true. A very small *p*-value (e.g. <0.001) is hardly affected by several comparisons, but adjusting less extreme *p*-values in this way could over-inflate them, and a real effect could be missed.

It may be preferable instead to present the unadjusted *p*-values, with a suitable note of caution if they are just below 0.05, and report 97.5% confidence intervals for say 2–3 comparisons, or 99% intervals for ≥3 comparisons, because they provide more conservative estimates of the range of the true effect (wider intervals).

Other methods for dealing with multiple endpoints include the **Holmberg** or **Hochberg procedures** (they can handle correlated endpoints), and **gate-keeping strategies** such as a **fixed sequence/sequential testing** approach (Section 5.12, page 74).[15, 16]

Gatekeeping strategies involve ordering or ranking endpoints or comparisons, and then performing statistical significance tests *in turn*. This is illustrated in Figure 7.6 using a hypothetical trial for type 2 diabetes and a fixed-sequence method. The ranking (ordering) of endpoints is crucial and influenced by which one is likely to show the greatest effect and whether the expected number of events would be large enough to lead to statistical significance and clinical relevance/value. This is often not easy to do.

Each 'box' in Figure 7.6 represents a statistical test for an endpoint. Claims that the treatment is effective for an endpoint should only be made if the *p*-value is <0.05.

• Basic principle: as long as each endpoint (or analysis) is statistically significant, the 5% error rate can be 'passed along' to the next analysis in the sequence. As soon as $p \geq 0.05$ the allowed 5% is used up, and none is left for subsequent analyses on the list.

• Advantages: 0.05 error rate can be used for each sample size for each analysis, so this approach does not increase the study size unlike e.g. Bonferroni methods; and claims can be made about several major outcome measures.

• Disadvantage: investigators have to pre-specify the ordering which they must get right in order to maximise the number of claims they can make.

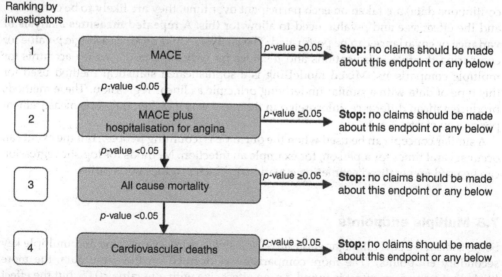

Figure 7.6 Illustration of a gatekeeping strategy using a fixed sequence method (sometimes called sequential or hierarchical testing). The ranking must be pre-specified in the trial protocol. MACE: fatal or non-fatal myocardial infarction or stroke.

Table 7.5 Example of hierarchical (sequential) testing in a clinical trial where several endpoints achieved statistical significance in the ranking. Source: Nissen et al.[17]

Ranking	Endpoints (HR and 95%CI)	P value	Objective
1	Cardiovascular (CV) death, nonfatal myocardial infarction (MI), nonfatal stroke, coronary vascularisation (0.87, 0.79–0.96)	P = 0.004	Achieved
2	CV death, nonfatal MI, nonfatal stroke (0.85, 0.76–0.96)	P = 0.006	Achieved
3	Fatal or nonfatal MI (0.77, 0.66–0.91)	P = 0.002	Achieved
4	Coronary vascularisation (0.81, 0.72–0.92)	P = 0.001	Achieved
5	Fatal or nonfatal stroke (0.85, 0.67–1.07)	P = 0.16	Failed
6	CV death (1.04, 0.88–1.24)		Failed
7	All-cause mortality (1.03, 0.90–1.18)		Failed

In a trial of bempedoic acid vs placebo for people who are statin intolerant,[17] the pre-specified ordering of the major endpoints and corresponding p-values and conclusions are shown in Table 7.5. This allowed major conclusions (claims) to be made for four endpoints (all of which appeared in the abstract of the journal article).

However, in another trial that used sequential testing (canagliflozin vs placebo for people with type 2 diabetes)[5] all-cause mortality was placed too high up as the second ranked endpoint and this objective failed because HR was 0.90 with p-value=0.24. Statistical testing had to stop with this endpoint, even though there was an apparent benefit for the fourth- and fifth-ranked endpoints below it, which were cardiovascular death and hospitalisation for heart failure (the 95%CIs excluded the no effect value).

7.9 Dealing with missing outcome data

It is always best to avoid missing data in the first place. When there are missing data, the main concern is whether the observed effect sizes are substantially under- or overestimated if the analyses are only based on non-missing data (i.e. biased). There are three general categories of missing data:

- **Missing completely at random**: the missing data do not depend on any factor (including the trial interventions), therefore participants with missing data have similar characteristics as those without missing data.
- **Missing at random**: the missing data depend on a factor that is unrelated to the trial interventions. For example, males could be more likely than females to have missing data, but this is acceptable as long as the effect of the treatment does not vary by sex.
- **Not missing at random**: the missing data are influenced by the trial interventions. For example, suppose the endpoint is quality of life (QoL); a new therapy can lead to serious side effects. More patients suffer adverse events with the new therapy than the controls, making them too ill to complete the QoL assessments, and these could have worse QoL scores had they been measured. Ignoring these patients will therefore overestimate the benefit of the new treatment on QoL.

The first two categories are generally not an issue, and analyses excluding those missing data might still be valid, but with fewer participants (or data) statistical significance could be missed.

The general approach to handling missing data is through **imputation**: missing data are estimated and then included in the analyses along with the non-missing data.[18,19]

This is referred to as **sensitivity analyses**. There are several methods for imputation, but one approach is to have conservative (occasionally extreme) assumptions, that try to bias the data away from having favourable results in the new treatment group.[#] This is because the findings and conclusions are more reliable if the main results are not substantially changed by such assumptions. For example, in the new treatment group we can assume missing data are similar to non-missing data from the controls. **Last observation carried forward (LOCF)** takes the last known value for a participant to use for later missing time points. But this assumes the outcome remains constant, and can be problematic if there is a long time gap between the last known value and the missing value. LOCF can overestimate the benefit of a new treatment and should be avoided unless it can be shown to be a valid method for a particular trial.

Another method called **multiple imputation** is more sophisticated. It uses *several* variables (e.g. the baseline factors and the treatment grouping), and constructs a model between these and the outcome measure, thus allowing for correlations between factors. The model is then used to estimate missing values for the outcome measure, and the analysis produces an effect size. The model can be used to provide different estimates of the missing values, and another estimate of effect is produced; this is repeated many times, e.g. 100. The final effect size is found by combining all 100 estimates. Multiple imputation can be performed for any simple test (e.g. t-test) or regression (linear, logistic and Cox).

The imputation methods above do not allow for 'not missing at random'. Statistical methods that can do this are more complex (e.g. **estimating-equation** or **multiple imputation by chained equation** methods), and require various assumptions to be made about the data.

7.10 Translational research[20,21]

Many trials evaluate biomarkers and imaging markers (see page 12).

Simple correlative analyses can be done between the marker and outcomes (e.g. the association between lipid levels and the risk of cardiovascular disease), using multivariable regression methods that allow for several baseline demographic and disease factors.

Randomised trials that use biomarkers to direct treatments (e.g. multiple experimental therapies Figure 5.2d, page 63) may not be sufficiently powered for evaluating *individual* treatments, therefore descriptive analyses or Bayesian statistics could be used to determine whether some therapies are effective but others are not. This would have to be done with care, and considering several efficacy endpoints, to avoid rejecting a therapy that is truly beneficial.

Similarly, there are issues for randomised basket trials (e.g. Figure 4.5, page 47) in which the same treatment is given to patients with different subtypes of a disorder (e.g. different cancer types), but they all have the same biomarker. Analyses can be performed for all patients but also each subtype separately, although the number of patients in some individual subtypes may be too small to make any meaningful conclusion about whether the new therapy is effective or not for these particular patients. Again, descriptive and Bayesian statistics might help.

In both phase II and III trials, exploratory analyses of multiple biomarkers at the end of the study might help explain why a new treatment is only effective in some people and

---

[#] For superiority trials, use assumptions to try to make the effect size smaller; for non-inferiority trials use assumptions to try to make the treatment inferior to the control group.

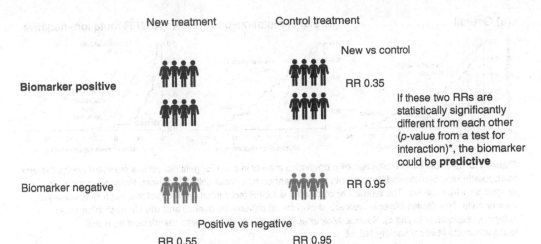

Figure 7.7 Illustration of the difference between a prognostic and predictive biomarker. RR (relative risk; but could also be hazard ratio or odds ratio) is for an outcome that is bad (e.g. death or disease event). Patient and disease characteristics should be similar between the New treatment and control group (due to randomisation) but possibly different when comparing biomarker-positive and -negative participants (multivariable regression analyses can allow for this). * Same test as in Box 7.3.

not others, especially if the overall effect size is small or modest. Two common goals are to see whether a biomarker is **predictive** or **prognostic** (Figure 7.7). They involve fundamentally different comparisons.

Personalised medicine is based on **predictive markers**, where the choice of treatment for a person depends on their biomarker status: a new therapy is only effective in some people, not all. If the effect sizes are similar (and interaction p-value>0.05), this means that the marker is not clinically useful: so just give the new therapy to everyone.

Figure 7.8 is an example of a predictive marker in oncology.[22] Among all trial patients, the effect of gefitinib is moderate (HR 0.74). Importantly, the Kaplan–Meier curves cross each other, which sometimes indicates an underlying predictive marker. When the data are divided according to EGFR mutation status, patients whose tumour is EGFR-positive have a large benefit when given gefitinib (HR for progressing or dying is 0.48, so risk is decreased), but those whose tumour is EGFR-negative actually have a detrimental effect from gefitinib (HR is 2.85, risk is increased by almost threefold). Notably, the curves do not cross anymore. The test for interaction p-value is <0.0001 (HR 0.48 is highly statistically different from 2.85). The clinical impact is that only EGFR-positive patients should receive gefitinib, and those who are EGFR-negative patients have standard chemotherapy, and this became recommended routine practice.

For a **prognostic marker**, interest is whether it can be used to forecast[#] a person's outcome or prognosis, regardless of treatment or among people given the same treatment.[23, 24] Figure 7.9 is an example (the biomarker is number of circulating tumour cells in blood).[25] The Kaplan-Meier curves (left figure) indicate how well the marker correlates

---

[#] A common term used was 'predicting' a person's outcome, but a predictive marker now has a different definition, as outlined above.

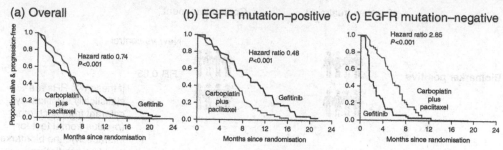

Figure 7.8 Example of an evaluation of a predictive marker in a trial of gefitinib versus standard chemotherapy (carboplatin plus pemetrexed) for patients with advanced non-small cell lung cancer. Primary endpoint is progression-free survival. The biomarker of interest is EGFR (epidermal growth factor receptor) assessed in cancer cells. The Kaplan-Meier curves are shown for all patients (a. overall) and then in each biomarker subgroup separately (b and c). Source: Mok et al.[22] / figure reproduced with permission from the Massachusetts Medical Society/NEJM.

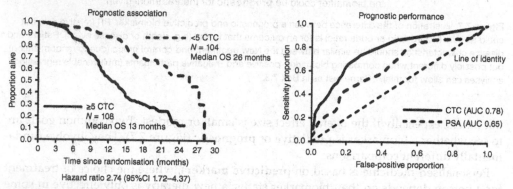

Figure 7.9 Example of evaluating a prognostic marker in a trial of patients with metastatic castration-resistant prostate cancer. The primary endpoint is overall survival. CTC: circulating tumour cells at baseline, PSA: prostate-specific antigen, AUC: area under the curve (the closer to 1, the better the marker). The left-hand figure shows the prognostic *association* between CTC and overall survival; the right-hand figure (receiver operator characteristic [ROC] curve) shows prognostic *performance* for two-year survival. The ROC curve is derived by examining sensitivity and false-positive proportion at each CTC count. Figures were created using approximate data points from the published curves.[25]

with overall survival: patients who had ≥5 circulating tumour cells (per 7.5 mL blood) had a much worse survival than those with <5 cells. A multivariable Cox regression analysis produced an adjusted hazard ratio of 2.74 for ≥5 versus <5 cells, allowing for potential confounding factors (e.g. age, ethnicity, prostate-specific antigen, performance status) as these may not be balanced between patients who had ≥5 or <5 circulating cells.

Measures like hazard ratio (odds ratio and relative risk) only reflect the strength of association (here, HR = 2.74 is a strong association). They do not indicate the clinical utility (performance) of the marker. This is shown using a receiver operator characteristic (ROC) curve (Figure 7.9) and key performance measures are:

Sensitivity: the percentage of people who are marker positive among all those who died by two years (i.e. had the event of interest).

False-positive rate (proportion): the percentage of people who are marker positive among all those who were alive at two years (i.e. did not have the event).

Excellent prognostic markers have sensitivity close to 100% and false-positive rate close to 0%.

Specificity is 1 minus the false-positive proportion.

The aim is to use the prognostic marker to identify those who die (have the event of interest) later, in order to act before with some preventive therapy or be monitored more closely. But also to minimise the number of people who do not die (do not have the event of interest) but are flagged as marker-positive and may then have preventive therapies or closer monitoring unnecessarily. The ROC curve for a useless marker would lie along the line of identity, so the area under the curve is 0.5 (sensitivity is the same as false-positive rate, so predicting a person's outcome is the same as chance). The better the performance of the marker the higher the ROC curve above the line of identity (and area under the curve gets closer to 1.0). In Figure 7.9, reading off the ROC curve, CTC count has sensitivity of ~60% and false-positive rate of ~20%, which appears to be a good but not striking performance. In Figure 7.9, the performance of CTC count is higher than for PSA, using the area under the curves (0.78 vs. 0.65). There are also statistical methods to compare the areas.

Investigators should carefully consider the clinical consequences for participants with and without the event of interest when they have marker-positive results. This can be done by applying observed values of sensitivity and false-positive rate, and also outlining what happens to those with an event who are marker-negative (i.e. missed).

Sensitivity, false-positive rate and the prevalence (or incidence) of the event (e.g. death) can be combined into positive predictive value (PPV): the percentage who have the event of interest only among those who are biomarker positive (the higher the PPV the better the marker).

Sometimes, multivariable regression models can include several prognostic factors including the biomarkers in order to build a **prognostic model** (which is also evaluated using ROC curves). Participants in a clinical trial dataset can be split (e.g. 1:1, 1:2 or 2:1) into a training set and internal validation set. The training set is used to develop the model and obtain parameters from a regression analysis. These parameters are then applied to the validation set from which sensitivity and false-positive rates are observed, to assess prognostic performance. An external validation set would come from a completely different source and also used to estimate performance measures.

There is often a misunderstanding that a prognostic factor that is well correlated with an outcome also means that it has good prognostic performance. However, the strength of the correlation (association) has to be very large in order for the performance to be good enough to be clinically useful.[26]

Developing biomarkers

It is important that the markers are measured reliably (e.g. validated assays), especially if they are used as part of the trial eligibility criteria or the primary or key secondary outcome measures. Newly developed markers may be best measured at qualified central laboratories. Unexpected lack of effects of a treatment on a biomarker may be due to the use of unvalidated markers (including assays and reagents), rather than a genuine lack of a biological effect.

Using markers and assays already available in routine practice are ideal because they are already tested and validated, as long as they are applied to situations that they are licensed for. A central laboratory is unlikely to be needed. When investigators develop their own marker (assay) they should consider the following:

- The biological rationale for the marker.
- Analytical validity, e.g. it measures the target of interest, it allows/overcomes noise or cross reactivity, and there is specification of sample quality and storage/processing requirements.
- Clinical validity, e.g. good marker performance using sensitivity and specificity, and internal and external validation of marker performance using independent datasets.
- Clinical utility, e.g. cost-effectiveness, how easy the sample processing, posting and storage requirements are when used routinely across multiple institutions, and whether patients and clinicians understand the marker result and its consequences.

References

1. Petrie A, Sabine C. *Medical Statistics at a Glance*. 4th edn, Wiley-Blackwell, 2019.
2. Kirkwood B, Sterne J. *Essential Medical Statistics*. 3rd edn, Wiley-Blackwell, 2019.
3. Lovell K, Cox D, Haddock G *et al*. Telephone administered cognitive behaviour therapy for treatment of obsessive compulsive disorder: randomised controlled non-inferiority trial. *BMJ* 2006; **333**:883–887.
4. Pfeffer MA, Claggett B, Diaz R *et al*.; ELIXA Investigators. Lixisenatide in patients with type 2 diabetes and acute coronary syndrome. *N Engl J Med* 2015; **373**(23):2247–2257.
5. Neal B, Perkovic V, Mahaffey KW *et al*.; CANVAS Program Collaborative Group. Canagliflozin and cardiovascular and renal events in type 2 diabetes. *N Engl J Med* 2017; **377**(7):644–665.
6. Marso SP, Bain SC, Consoli A *et al*.; SUSTAIN-6 Investigators. Semaglutide and cardiovascular outcomes in patients with type 2 diabetes. *N Engl J Med* 2016; **375**(19):1834–1844
7. Shitara K, Bang YJ, Iwasa S *et al*.; DESTINY-Gastric01 Investigators. Trastuzumab deruxtecan in previously treated HER2-positive gastric cancer. *N Engl J Med* 2020; **382**(25):2419–2430.
8. Cuzick J. Forest plots and the interpretation of subgroups. *Lancet* 2005; **365**:1308.
9. Dehbi H, Hackshaw A. Investigating subgroup effects in randomized clinical trials. *J Clin Oncol* 2016; **35**:253–254.
10. Collins R, MacMahon S. Reliable assessment of the effects of treatment on mortality and major morbidity, I: clinical trials. *Lancet* 2001; **357**(9253):373–380.
11. MRC Vitamin Study Research Group. Prevention of neural tube defects: results of the MRC vitamin study. *Lancet* 1991; **338**:132–137.
12. Lopes RD, Heizer G, Aronson R *et al*.; AUGUSTUS Investigators. Antithrombotic therapy after acute coronary syndrome or PCI in atrial fibrillation. *N Engl J Med* 2019; **380**(16):1509–1524.
13. Bland JM, Kerry SM. The intracluster correlation coefficient in cluster randomisation. *BMJ* 1998; **316**:1455–1460.
14. Hooper R, Forbes A, Hemming K, Takeda A, Beresford L. Analysis of cluster randomised trials with an assessment of outcome at baseline. *BMJ* 2018; **360**:k1121.

15. Multiple Endpoints in Clinical Trials Guidance for Industry. Center for Drug Evaluation and Research (CDER). Food and Drug Administration. October 2022. https://www.fda.gov/regulatory-information/search-fda-guidance-documents/multiple-endpoints-clinical-trials-guidance-industry.

16. Dmitrienko A, D'Agostino RB Sr. Multiplicity considerations in clinical trials. *N Engl J Med* 2018; **378**(22):2115–2122.

17. Nissen SE, Lincoff AM, Brennan D *et al.*; CLEAR Outcomes Investigators. Bempedoic acid and cardiovascular outcomes in statin-intolerant patients. *N Engl J Med* 2023; **388**(15):1353–1364.

18. Little RJ, D'Agostino R, Cohen ML *et al.* The prevention and treatment of missing data in clinical trials. *N Engl J Med* 2012; **367**(14):1355–1360.

19. Li P, Stuart EA, Allison DB. Multiple imputation: a flexible tool for handling missing data. *JAMA* 2015; **314**(18):1966–1967.

20. Freidlin B, Korn EL. Biomarker enrichment strategies: matching trial design to biomarker credentials. *Nat Rev Clin Oncol* 2014; **11**(2):81–90.

21. Polley MY, Freidlin B, Korn EL *et al.* Statistical and practical considerations for clinical evaluation of predictive biomarkers. *J Natl Cancer Inst* 2013; **105**(22):1677–1683.

22. Mok TS, Wu YL, Thongprasert S *et al.* Gefitinib or carboplatin-paclitaxel in pulmonary adenocarcinoma. *N Engl J Med* 2009; **361**(10):947–957.

23. Pajouheshnia R, Groenwold RHH, Peelen LM *et al.* When and how to use data from randomised trials to develop or validate prognostic models. *BMJ* 2019; **365**:l2154.

24. Bonnett LJ, Snell KIE, Collins GS, Riley RD. Guide to presenting clinical prediction models for use in clinical settings. *BMJ* 2019; **365**:l737.

25. Goldkorn A, Ely B, Quinn DI *et al.* Circulating tumor cell counts are prognostic of overall survival in SWOG S0421: a phase III trial of docetaxel with or without atrasentan for metastatic castration-resistant prostate cancer. *J Clin Oncol* 2014; **32**(11):1136–1142.

26. Wald NJ, Hackshaw AK, Frost CD. When can a risk factor be used as a worthwhile screening test? *BMJ* 1999; **319**(7224):1562–1565.

CHAPTER 8

Commercial trials of medicinal products; other types of interventions; health economic analysis

This chapter provides an overview of how new therapies are licensed for use in humans and then evaluated before being implemented into routine care; some general comments about designing and conducting trials of interventions other than medicinal products; and a brief outline of health economic analyses.

8.1 Commercial trials of medicines (drugs)#

Commercially sponsored clinical trials (mainly pharmaceutical companies) play a key role in improving health, especially for treating advanced or hard-to-treat disorders. Figure 8.1 shows the typical pathway from clinical trials to post-marketing (real-world evidence) studies. Traditionally, the pathway took many years but there are now ways to reduce this, e.g. merging different clinical phases into the same protocol (Phase II/III).

The two main types of approvals are **regulatory** and **health technology assessment (market access)**. They have different and overlapping functions (Figure 8.2). Table 8.1 shows examples of organisations that perform these reviews in several countries.

When planning one or more pivotal trials it is often worth seeking advice from these agencies, particularly on the design, choice of the control group and primary outcome measures, and (where applicable) the non-inferiority margin. Although the advice is not binding and the recommendations do not guarantee that a future regulatory or market access application will be successful, it can minimise major criticisms. However, sponsors should be willing to make changes to their design if proposed, and if they are not then they should reconsider whether requesting advice is going to be helpful after all. Sponsors can also get independent advice on trial design from specialist clinical and non-clinical experts in the disorder of interest (key opinion leaders), and this can be used to support the final choice of design when being submitted for approval later on.

Both small and large pharmaceutical companies face challenges over modern clinical trials (Box 8.1).

Small companies may have particular resource challenges including lack of in-house clinical trial expertise, limited infrastructure and ultimately limited funding. They often rely on **contract research organisations** or hire consultants. This can mean that relatively short trials are preferred, if possible. Many small biotech companies have been created,

---

Several aspects also apply to some medical devices.

A Concise Guide to Clinical Trials, Second Edition. Allan Hackshaw.
© 2024 John Wiley & Sons Ltd. Published 2024 by John Wiley & Sons Ltd.

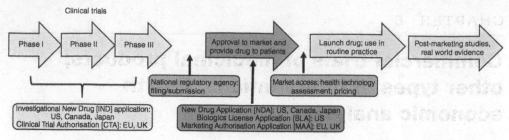

Figure 8.1 Overview of the process of drug development from clinical trials to launch and real-world evidence.

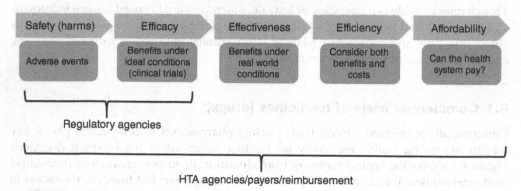

Figure 8.2 Overview of what regulatory and health technology assessment (HTA) agencies/payers examine.

Table 8.1 Examples of national regulatory and health technology assessment (HTA)/reimbursement agencies.

Location	Regulatory agency	HTA/reimbursement agency
US	Food & Drug Administration (FDA)	Several, e.g. the Agency for Healthcare Research and Quality (AHRQ); Medicare, Medicaid and private insurance providers
Canada	Health Canada	Canadian Agency for Drugs and Technologies in Health (CADTH)
Europe	European Medicines Association (EMA)	EUnetHTA* (EU HTA regulation 2021/2282)
UK	Medicines and Healthcare products Regulatory Agency (MHRA)	National Institute for Health and Care Excellence (NICE)
Germany	Federal Institute for Drugs and Medical Devices (BfArM) and the Paul-Ehrlich-Institut	Institute for Quality and Efficiency in Healthcare (IQWiG) Gemeinsamer Bundesausschuss (G-BA)
France	National Agency for the Safety of Medicines and Health Products (ANSM)	Haute Autorité de Santé (HAS)
Japan	Pharmaceuticals and Medical Devices Agency (PMDA)	Ministry of Health, Labour and Welfare (MHLW)
Australia	Therapeutic Goods Administration (TGA)	Pharmaceutical Benefits Advisory Committee (PBAC)
India	Drugs Controller General of India (DCGI); Central Drugs Standard Control Organisation (CDSCO)	Health Technology Assessment India (HTAIn), under the Department of Health and Research
China	National Medical Products Administration (NMPA)	National Healthcare Security Administration (NHSA)

* Collaboration between several individual HTA agencies from EU countries.

Box 8.1 Potential challenges with clinical trials

• Need to satisfy several organisations with different remits (regulators, HTA/payers, national guideline bodies, clinicians and health service managers, patients/public)
• Trials are expensive (e.g. large infrastructure of staff, multicentre, multicountry)
• Too many eligibility criteria (not representative of the 'real-world')
• Too complex (e.g. many endpoints, procedures, sub-studies)
• When current treatments are already very effective, larger trials are needed to show superiority of new therapies that can have only small/modest benefits.
• Head-to-head trials (non-inferiority) are sometimes expected and are large.
• Trials of chronic disorders need long treatment duration and/or long follow-up.
• Need to find biomarkers to target subgroups to increase chance of finding an effective therapy.
• Deciding which point of the disease pathway to focus on (e.g. treatments for Alzheimer's disease could have larger effects when given to patients with early symptoms, not at a later stage, but then many people who would never progress could be over-treated).

---

sometimes focussing on rare disorders that are hard to treat, using new technologies, targeted therapies (for a particular genetic or marker abnormality) or repurposed products. These trials tend to be single-arm and relatively small. However, striking efficacy results in areas of unmet need could lead to regulatory and market access approvals, despite the trial design limitations.

Licencing and marketing authorisation

Without a **licence** or **market authorisation** no manufacturer can advertise, provide or sell a new pharmaceutical product (and some medical devices) to patients, clinicians and healthcare providers except within a research study for which explicit regulatory approval must be obtained (see Chapter 10) or under special circumstances (e.g. an early access to medicines scheme). This is required for every country, though in Europe the EMA can grant a single approval for all member states.

A national regulatory agency has to be satisfied that a new drug (on its own or in combination with standard therapies) has benefits for patients/public with acceptable side effects. The review is typically done by a panel of clinicians, chemists, pharmacologists, toxicologists, pharmacovigilance experts, statisticians and other specialist scientists/experts. They review:

• Pre-clinical studies and early and (where available) late phase clinical trials
• Efficacy, study quality, and reliability of treatment effects
• Harms, including incidence, severity and how easily treatable
• Manufacturing quality and recommendations for the drug label.

For drugs intended for children and adolescents, the sponsor develops a **Paediatric Investigation Plan (PIP)** in Europe or a **Pediatric Study Plan (PSP)** in the US for the phase I to III trials to ensure that sufficient data are collected on efficacy and safety.

For many disorders, especially chronic disorders, at least two trials of the same intervention should be done (e.g. in different geographical locations) to ensure that the therapy is effective and the magnitude of the benefit is reliably estimated. This may be required by regulatory agencies and payers. However, for uncommon/rare disorders, there may only be a single randomised trial, and in some cases, only single-arm trials.

Box 8.2 Pathways to obtain a licence or marketing authorisation for a new drug by the FDA and EMA (details may change over time)

US FDA	EU EMA
Standard review	Standard review
Accelerated approval	Conditional marketing authorisation
	Exceptional circumstances
Fast track	Accelerated review or PRIority MEdicines scheme (PRIME)
Breakthrough designation	
Priority review	

Standard reviews typically take about 10–12 months from the time of submission to a decision by the regulatory agency. **Expedited pathways** involve shorter review times (2–8 months), and are intended for disorders with unmet medical needs (e.g. no currently approved or effective therapy), rare disorders or subtypes, the new drug represents a major advance in treatment or has a major impact on patients or public health, or the treatment is highly innovative.

There are standard and various expedited pathways for granting a licence (Box 8.2). For accelerated approval and conditional authorisation, the regulatory agency provides a licence using preliminary data (e.g. surrogate markers, single-arm trials) and may often then request evidence to be provided by further studies (e.g. hard endpoints such as overall survival and randomised studies) in order to either grant a full licence or withdraw the initial licence after reviewing the additional data. If the safety profile is not well understood yet, the drug label (prescription) contains 'black box' warnings with regard to potentially serious side effects.

Special attention can be given to orphan drugs for rare disorders (e.g. where the prevalence/incidence is <5 per 10,000) that are life threatening or severely debilitating.

Market access (reimbursement)

Healthcare providers (payers) have limited resources. 'Market access' represents the process by which a new drug, medical device, or sometimes a new combination of licenced drugs, is made available in routine practice, so that all eligible patients have access to it and that it is affordable to the payer. Market access covers three linked areas[1]:

- **Health technology assessment (HTA)**: comprehensive evidence reviews, Figure 8.3.
- **Pricing and reimbursement (P&R)**: achieving an optimal price from the healthcare provider.
- **Formulary** (pharmacy): getting the drug placed on national lists of approved medicines, which includes information about dosing, contraindications, and side effects.

The different remits of regulatory and HTA agencies (Figure 8.2) can sometimes be a challenge to sponsors (manufacturers), who may have to conduct two or more clinical trials to satisfy both. HTA organisations may prefer head-to-head trials in some situations, where

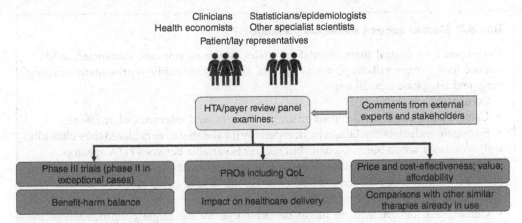

Figure 8.3 Typical constitution of an HTA review panel and what evidence they consider before approving or rejecting a drug for routine use and reimbursement. PRO, patient-reported outcomes; QoL, health-related quality of life.

a new drug is compared with a current standard of care used in that geographical region (e.g. a competitor's drug within the same class). There is also variation in how HTA agencies from different countries review evidence.[1]

The Joint Clinical Assessment (JCA) is associated with an EU regulation that replaces the separate evaluation of clinical trial data by each EU country-specific HTA agency with a single harmonised assessment of relative effectiveness and safety. EUnetHTA has developed guidance documents on this. The JCA is non-binding and each EU member state makes its own value judgements and pricing and reimbursement decisions. However, the JCA report should be considered and be part of the documentation that each member state uses for decision-making.

Heath Technology Assessment (HTA)/payer/reimbursement review

Figure 8.3 illustrates the typical membership and functions of a review panel for HTA. The review may be performed by a payer or another organisation on behalf of the payer. The payer will often follow the advice of the organisation who conducted the assessment but, in some cases, will make a contrary conclusion and decision. Ultimately, the payer negotiates an acceptable price with the manufacturer.

Strong trial design (evidence), large treatment effects (benefits that far exceed current standard therapies), first or second to market, and unmet need are expected to be associated with premium pricing. Occasionally, the HTA review panel focus on a subgroup, and may even restrict the approval to this. Sponsors (manufacturers) need to be mindful of the problems with such analyses (Box 7.4, page 114).

Market access evidence package

A market access evidence package can be developed early (Box 8.3), acknowledging that it is unusual for a single study to provide all of the information required by decision-makers. A market access strategy includes deciding where to launch the drug first. The choice of countries (markets) can depend on several factors:
- the incidence of the disorder and expected trends over time
- use of competitor drugs in each of those countries and the expected percentage market share of the new drug

---

Box 8.3 Market access evidence package

Developed by a clinical team, regulatory affairs, health economists, statistician, medical science liaison representatives, market access, and patient/public representatives; using early and late phase clinical trials.

Considerations are:

- Using clinical and HTA-accepted efficacy endpoints, and relevant QoL measures.
- Surrogate endpoints can be accepted, especially if validated or considered to be clinically well-correlated with a hard outcome, but success is variable between HTA agencies.
- Ensuring that the comparator therapy is relevant to current clinical practice. In addition to RCTs, indirect comparisons with other standards of care could be planned using real world data (see Section 9.3, page 159).
- Clinical trial design features might be influenced by the target countries where the drug/medical device would be launched first/early (i.e. what those HTAs expect in terms of endpoints and comparator).
- Are there additional efficiencies or savings in healthcare delivery by using the new drug/medical device (e.g. fewer side effects therefore fewer hospital stays/lower costs of treating the events)?
- Are there resource impacts on healthcare delivery (e.g. nurses required to give injections of the new drug in clinic, whereas the current standard of care involves taking a tablet at home)?
- Does the healthcare system need to implement anything new to administer the new drug/medical device (the cost of which may need to be added to the drug price)?
- Whether there are evidence gaps in the pivotal clinical trials that can be obtained from observational real-world data instead (e.g. adherence, QoL, patient satisfaction).

- reference pricing (drugs are grouped according to therapeutic class and pricing may be limited to the price of the cheapest drug, one of the cheapest in that class, or the average price across selected countries)
- the likelihood of receiving approval from particular HTAs given the class of drug and disorder, from past experience.

Some countries (e.g. Japan) may expect to see data on local participants in an HTA submission, therefore international clinical trials can aim to recruit a certain minimum number in such countries (e.g. 30–50). This does not mean that the trial is powered for this particular cohort, but rather that some data can be used to show consistency in efficacy and safety with the overall results. It may also be possible to use real-world data from specific countries instead of including them in the pivotal trials. The design and statistical plan of these could be made upfront when the clinical trial is being developed.

Investigators should aim to understand the potentially different standards of background care between countries and whether this can affect the efficacy results. In some cases, there may be genuine biological (genetic) differences that lead to varying response to a new therapy, which could be explored by descriptive analyses.

In addition to the evidence package (with its focus on efficacy and harms), it might also be worthwhile to undertake research into what other things might matter to current and future patients (or the public) and their treating clinicians:

- Impact on a person's ability to function physically and socially, and work
- Any inconvenience to patients/public in order to access the therapy
- Impact on carers

Patient advocacy groups should be involved and this can be used as supporting evidence in an HTA submission that includes the clinical trial evidence.

For example, consider a three-arm non-inferiority trial of HIV treatment that aimed to replace one or two of the standard drugs with alternative drugs that have fewer side effects. One experimental arm involved replacing efavirenz with dolutegravir; and the other experimental arm involved replacing tenofovir disoproxil fumarate and efavirenz with tenofovir alafenamide fumarate and dolutegravir.[2] The primary outcome was viral load <50 copies per ml and the trial objective was successfully achieved for both experimental arms, i.e. the percentage of people who had a low/undetectable viral load in these groups was high and similar to the control group, and there were significantly fewer high grade adverse events as expected. However, both experimental groups had a weight gain of, on average, 3–6 kg by 48 weeks. Many years ago, focus was on reducing the high mortality and morbidity associated with HIV progressing to AIDS; weight gain would not have been a priority. However, in many places the majority of people *now* with HIV live a normal life with adequate treatment, so weight gain among these is likely to be an issue; particularly given their relatively young age group, the risk of cardiovascular disease, and the possibility that the weight gain increases with longer treatment duration. This example should encourage sponsors to ensure that their market access evidence package goes beyond the standard efficacy and harms outcomes, to cover the deliverability and appeal/acceptability of the new intervention.

Clinical trial design

Clinical trial design features were covered in Chapters 4 and 5, and the same principles apply to studies to be used for regulatory approval and market access. The design can influence when and how a new drug is launched (Figure 8.4). Major limitations of the design features can lead to rejection of the drug or medical device by an HTA.

Choosing a comparator could involve considering what the future standards of care might be in order to 'future proof' the trial (perhaps as a second control arm). Investigators can look at trends in uptake of approved competitor therapies, likely market share in the future, and ongoing trials of therapies that might become standards of care by the time the sponsor's own planned trial finishes.

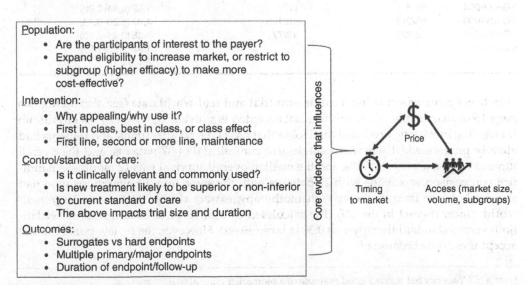

Figure 8.4 Clinical trial design features can influence market access.

Co-primary or multiple primary/major outcome measures (Section 5.12, page 74), including those that consist of a combination of hard and surrogate endpoints, may strengthen the evidence because the trial would be powered for several outcomes. It is also possible to submit data on one endpoint for an early regulatory licence (e.g. a surrogate marker that is analysed earlier), and the second endpoint (e.g. hard outcome) submitted later for full/standard approval. This staged approach could allow the therapy to be marketed earlier under certain conditions.

Supporting evidence: systematic reviews (meta-analyses) and real-world evidence

Given the variation in how HTAs review evidence, due to different healthcare systems, it can be difficult to design 1–2 clinical trials that can satisfy everyone. Supporting evidence can come from other sources, and the HTA review panel will determine the reliability of these and therefore, whether they can contribute to the evaluation of a new therapy. Systematic reviews (meta-analysis) and indirect comparisons using real-world evidence are covered in Chapter 9, including their value and limitations. Sometimes, this evidence is successfully used, but other times it is rejected though approval may still be granted based on the clinical trial(s) alone.

Systematic review of randomised trials: an example of a successful application of a meta-analysis is seen in a submission to the German HTA (IQWiG), for the drug ocriplasmin for treating vitreomacular traction in adults (an eye disorder where the vitreous gel has an abnormally strong adhesion to the retina, causing defective vision).[3] The submitted evidence consisted of three relatively small trials, of which only one was statistically significant, but the pooled effect size showed a clear effect with strong evidence ($p = 0.001$); Table 8.2.

Table 8.2 Meta-analysis of three randomised trials of ocriplasmin for treating vitreomacular traction. An event is improvement in vision. Source: Adapted from IQWiG Reports[3].

| Trial ID | No. of events/No. of patients | | Relative risk of improvement in visual acuity (95%CI) |
	Ocriplasmin injection	Watchful waiting (sham/ placebo injection)	
TG-MV-004	6/13	2/7	1.62 (0.44–5.99)
TG-MV-006	63/210	16/105	1.97 (1.20–3.23)
TG-MV-007	58/226	12/77	1.65 (0.94–2.90)
Combined			1.82 (1.26–2.58)
			$P = 0.001$

Indirect comparison using a single-arm trial and real-world data (see also section 9.3 page 159): an example where this was not accepted is a review by the FDA[#] of erdafitinib for treating metastatic urothelial carcinoma that has *FGFR2/3* alterations, and patients had already progressed.[4] There was a single-arm clinical trial of 87 patients, and the overall tumour response rate was 32%, and the median overall survival was 12 months. An indirect comparison was made with 27 patients with the same tumour alterations who had standard-of-care immunotherapy/chemotherapy, extracted from Flatiron (a large real-world cancer dataset in the US). The calculated overall survival hazard ratio for erdafitinib versus standard therapy was 0.30 (a large effect). However, the review panel did not accept these data because of:

[#] Not a HTA agency but this is a good example of a biomarker clinical trial.

- Small number of comparator patients ($n = 27$)
- Uncertainty over dates of diagnosis for measuring survival time
- Incomplete/missing data (e.g. deaths)
- Unmeasured confounding factors
- Bias
  - ○ Trial patients came from academic medical centres
  - ○ Control patients came from community oncology clinics
- May not have captured all anti-cancer treatments (some patients were treated outside of the Flatiron network)

All of the above reasons are typical limitations of real-world data and why decision-makers, particularly HTA agencies, sometimes reject this evidence (despite their potential value). Nevertheless, the FDA still granted an accelerated approval for erdafitinib based on the clinical trial because of the poor prognosis in this patient group, and the efficacy results looked good.

There are examples where an indirect comparison using real-world data was used successfully, either for the main approval (e.g. avelumab for advanced Merkel cell carcinoma) or for a label expansion (e.g. palbociclib for males with advanced breast cancer, and blinatumomab for patients with acute lymphoblastic leukaemia with minimal residual disease).[5]

Sponsors (manufacturers) must either design their own reliable and high quality real-world data studies to avoid or minimise major methodological issues, or only use external data sources that are high quality. However, such studies should not replace RCTs when these are feasible.

See section 'Cell and gene therapy' (page 142) for an example where an HTA agency evaluated a single-arm trial alongside indirect evidence for a comparator therapy.

8.2 Other types of interventions

Numerous interventions can be used in medical care (prevention or treatment). The fundamental principles of design and analysis covered in Chapters 2–7 can be applied to any type: surgery, behavioural, alternative/complementary therapies (e.g. acupuncture), and radiotherapy or radioactive substances.

Screening and early detection uses imaging and biomarker tests to identify people with early stage disease that can be treated successfully or cured, or find those at high risk of a disorder to offer them preventive therapies. RCTs are often, but not always, needed to evaluate screening tests. The intervention being evaluated in a RCT is usually the combination of the screening test plus whatever therapies are given to screen-positives. Study outcome measures (sensitivity, false-positive rates and reduction/prevention of events) need to reflect clear and clinically meaningful impacts on patients or the public. They also need to reflect harms among false-positives (i.e. people who do/will not have the disorder of interest but they are screen-positive): unnecessary investigations or therapies that are harmful or expensive.

There are also randomised trials of implementation research, e.g. new processes or systems that aim to improve healthcare delivery, monitoring and efficiency. These are not always based on individuals but rather healthcare units, e.g. hospital wards, hospitals, and primary care practices, therefore cluster randomised trials are used.

Box 8.4 lists some key considerations of trials of selected different types of interventions. Unlike medicinal products that are manufactured in the same way, the delivery

Box 8.4 Some key considerations of trials of selected different types of interventions

Surgery	Radiotherapy (radioactive substances)	Behavioural (e.g. diet, exercise, lifestyle)
Established first step for many disorders (curative), and often used alone	Often used as add-on therapy, and can be given at several points on the treatment pathway	Often used to reduce symptoms or risk factors, or improve quality of life
Most trials are unblinded; others can only be single-blinded; the assessor could be blinded who is not the same surgeon who delivered the procedure	Most trials are unblinded; others can only be single-blinded; the assessor could be blinded	Most trials are unblinded; the assessor could be blinded
Often high adherence	Adherence might be affected if patients have to attend hospital many times per week or month	Might have high non-adherence, especially for complex interventions with long duration
Quality control is ideal but may be difficult. Surgeons can use different techniques and tools for the same operation, and the pre- and post-operative care can also influence outcomes.	Quality control/assurance is needed to ensure the therapy is delivered to the same high standard across several centres (but this can be arduous to do sometimes)	Interventions should be easy to follow ideally. For complex interventions (mixture of several components); it may not be easy to tell which items were effective or not.
Focus is often on short-term adverse effects and postoperative mortality (e.g. 30 days later)	Both short- and long-term adverse effects often matter (e.g. radiation fibrosis) Safety restrictions are needed for those who deliver radioactive therapies.	Usually, safe
Single centre trials may over-estimate benefit if it is an expert centre	Advanced radiotherapy techniques might only be available in a few centres (limiting trial accrual)	Participants may find it easy to access/use the intervention from the other trial arm (crossover)

of surgical techniques and behavioural interventions can vary, and so are difficult to standardise (this reflects real life).

Clinical trials can also compare therapies in current routine use, so there is essentially no concept of a control group (called **randomised comparative effectiveness trials**).

Surgical techniques[6-8]

Surgery has been the cornerstone of treatment for many disorders. This could involve major surgical operations using general anaesthesia or relatively minor procedures that can be performed under local anaesthetic. Advances in surgery (e.g. keyhole and robotics) have led to safer and less invasive procedures, but randomised trials are needed to ensure that efficacy is not compromised.

There are several issues specific to surgical trials. A common one is that although surgeons agree to participate in a randomised trial, they often do not have equipoise when faced with an individual patient and may choose or recommend what they consider to be the best treatment. Patients may also have a preference for one surgical procedure over another, especially if surgery is being compared with a non-surgical intervention such that patients choose the one that seems the most appealing. This may affect the generalisability of the results, and lead to slow accrual. It might be best to have very clear patient-facing materials, including simple videos, and a health professional who is not a surgeon (e.g. a research nurse) could provide most of the information and address queries by the patient and then take consent.

Most surgical trials cannot be blinded but, on occasion and where ethical, sham surgery can be used as the comparator. An example was a single-blind trial for osteoarthritis of the knee where patients were randomised to arthroscopic lavage, débridement or sham surgery (see page 11).[9] All trial patients were unaware of the procedure applied and all had skin scars. After the placebo effect had been accounted for there was no benefit from surgery.

Box 8.5 outlines two examples of complementary trials.[10, 11] The following are noted, and can apply to other surgical trials:

- They each took many years to recruit (80 participants for the severe hernia group 2011–2020, 196 participants for the moderate hernia group 2008–2019), despite having multiple centres. This might reflect the general difficulty in getting enough patients to agree to be randomised.
- Standard care could have changed during this time, but it should be the same in each group so may not affect the results.
- There were multiple surgeons across multiple sites, hence generalisable.
- Centres were required to demonstrate experience in performing FETO before joining. Surgeon experience could affect the success of the procedure.
- The trial of moderate hernia had two primary endpoints, and the trial of severe hernia used a group-sequential design to allow for several formal interim analyses; both are features of modern trials of drugs, showing that surgical studies can be similarly well-designed and conducted.
- The authors commented that they had no long-term outcome measures.

The example in Box 8.5 was a superiority trial. However, many 'new' surgical techniques are less invasive than current procedures so non-inferiority trials are required. The

---

Box 8.5 Example of two-phase III trials of surgery. Sources: Deprest et al.[10]; Deprest et al.[11]

Location: Multicentre and several countries

Participants: Pregnant women carrying a foetus with either a moderate or severe left diaphragmatic hernia; separate trials were done for each type

Intervention: Fetoscopic endoluminal tracheal occlusion (FETO, balloon insertion) performed 30–32 weeks gestation for the moderate hernia group, and 27–29 weeks for the severe hernia group

Control: Standard expectant care

Outcome measures: Infant survival at discharge from neonatal intensive care. The moderate hernia group also had survival without oxygen supplementation at 6 months of age (as a multiple primary endpoint).

Results: FETO was beneficial for severe hernia but there was insufficient benefit for moderate hernia and there were harms.

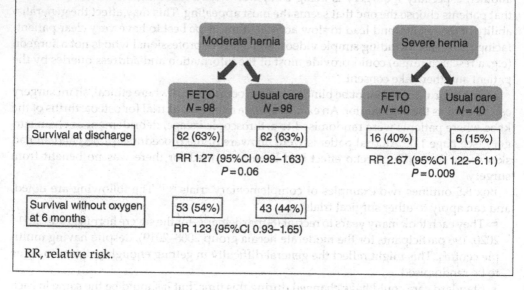

RR, relative risk.

---

surgical technique of interest is often already used in routine practice, which can make a randomised trial difficult to do.

The Laparoscopic Approach to Cervical Cancer (LACC) trial compared minimally invasive (conventional laparoscopic or robotic surgery) with standard open abdominal radical hysterectomy, in women with early stage cervical cancer.[12] In the trial design, the 4.5-year disease-free survival (DFS) rate was assumed to be 90% with standard surgery and the non-inferiority margin risk difference was −7.2 percentage points (i.e. a DFS rate down to 82.8% with minimal surgery was considered acceptable). Unexpectedly, the trial results were against minimal surgery, with a risk difference of −10.6 percentage points (95% CI −16.4 to −4.7); clearly exceeding the allowable margin, and considered an unacceptable loss in efficacy.

The Proximal Fracture of the Humerus Evaluation by Randomization (PROFHER) trial aimed to determine whether people who had a displaced shoulder fracture benefit from surgery (fracture fixation or humeral head replacement), compared to non-surgical management (sling immobilisation). It was a generally well-designed study, but notable points that can be applied to other surgical trials were: (i) an inclusion criterion was "clear indication for surgery", hence surgeons might have only selected patients for the trial with more favourable fractures; (ii) the average age of recruited patients was 66 so there may be some uncertainty over applying the trial results to young people who have complex fractures, (iii) the primary endpoint was the Oxford Shoulder Score that quantified patients' subjective assessment of pain and function but this score was not developed for people with traumatic events like fractures so may not reflect all relevant symptoms, and (iv) after randomisation 13% allocated to the surgical group did not have it but 2% allocated to the non-surgical group decided to have surgery after all, this clear imbalance in adherence could distort the intention-to-treat results.[13]

Radiotherapy and radioactive substances[14,15]

Radiotherapy (RT) is used for treating several disorders, and in particular cancer. About half of cancer patients receive RT at some point, and it can be used for any stage of disease. Conformal RT based on high-energy X-rays (photons) has been the standard method. However, there are more sophisticated approaches designed to deliver a higher dose of radiation but more focused on the affected tissue or organ and not the surrounding healthy tissue. These include intensity-modulated radiotherapy (IMRT), image-guided RT, stereotactic ablative body RT, stereotactic radiosurgery and proton beam therapy. There are also radiopharmaceuticals, in which patients swallow or are injected with a radioactive substance (e.g. radioactive iodine ablation for treating well-differentiated thyroid cancer).

RT trials have several aims, including RT dose de-escalation (non-inferiority trials) or dose-escalation (superiority trials), and the timing of RT. Further trial objectives can involve evaluating RT in combination with medicinal products; e.g. targeted cancer drugs and immunotherapies to minimise toxicity to healthy tissue and organs, and improve local tumour control and survival, compared with systemic drugs alone. Trials comparing RT with very different modalities (for example, surgery or oral drugs) can be difficult to recruit to because of the clear difference in treatment delivery.

Although the scientific rationale for a RT trial might be strong, acceptability by patients and adherence can be influenced by the following:

• What treatments they have had already (giving RT in addition to multiple other therapies may not appear worthwhile to patients)
• Number of visits to the clinic for the RT sessions by the patient and carer (travel and hotel costs).
• If patients are elderly, with comorbidities and fatigue, the frequency of travel may deter them from attending all sessions.
• Interruptions in RT can have a negative impact on relapse and survival, thus diluting the treatment effect.

Behavioural/lifestyle interventions[16,17]

Clinical trials of changing behaviours or lifestyles are particularly useful for chronic disorders to alleviate symptoms; reducing risk factors such as smoking or body weight; and preventing disorders such as cardiovascular disease. Box 8.4 outlines some main considerations.

Lack of blinding and the inability to measure adherence reliably can be major and unavoidable limitations. Complex interventions might have a good scientific rationale and people who agree to participate in a randomised trial might have high adherence, but investigators need to consider whether such interventions can be rolled out on a wide scale if shown to be positive in the trial.

Box 8.6 is an example of a lifestyle prevention trial, where the interventions were two diets.[18] The following are noted, and can apply to other behavioural change trials:

• The central study team were blinded to the interventions but the participants and the dieticians were not blinded

• The interventions had to be delivered by trained staff, and this involved a mixture of face-to-face and group sessions and telephone calls (at least 12 interactions each year). The interventions are actually the diet itself plus all of the contact sessions.

• This close level of contact helps to encourage adherence, which was relatively high in both trial groups throughout the study duration, though measured by self-completed questionnaires.

Box 8.6 Example of a lifestyle intervention trial. Source: Delgado-Lista et al.[18]/ figure reproduced with permission from Elsevier/The Lancet

Location: Single centre, Spain

Participants: People aged 20–75 years who have coronary heart disease

Intervention: Mediterranean diet, including extra-virgin olive oil provided for free

Control: Low-fat diet, including food packs rich in complex carbohydrates provided for free

Outcome measures: Major cardiovascular event.

Results: Hazard ratio 0.73 95% CI 0.55–0.97, $p = 0.03$

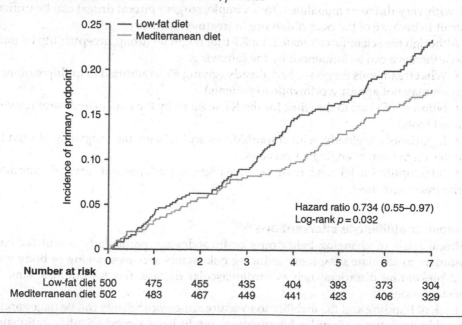

- The effect size and also the ability to deliver the Mediterranean diet in other places might not be considered generalisable given the relatively homogenous participant group in a location where the Mediterranean diet is already well known and accepted (single geographical location), and so there was high adherence during the trial.
- Each trial group would be aware of the intervention in the other group, and could switch if they wished.
- There was no control group that received nothing, even if this would reflect usual practice. Both arms of behavioural trials may need to appear sufficiently appealing to encourage participants to agree to take part.

The trial showed a clear and clinically worthwhile reduction in cardiovascular disease (27% reduction).Although it took about 3 years for a difference to be seen, the effect appeared to be maintained thereafter up to 7 years.

Medical devices[19–21]

There is a wide variety of medical devices. Simple devices such as elastic bandages would be considered low-risk and planned trials often do not require regulatory review and approval. Others are attached to the body externally and some are inserted or implanted internally, which may require an invasive surgical procedure. These may represent moderate- or high-risk devices. Investigators should always check whether a particular device planned for a clinical trial comes under national regulations or not. When they do, the studies are set up, conducted and monitored in a similar way as trials of medicinal drugs.

In the US, for example, medical device manufacturers must apply for and obtain an Individual Device Exemption (IDE) from the FDA in order to conduct a clinical trial in humans when the device is not yet approved for its intended use. A feasibility study focuses on collecting safety data from a small number of participants (typically <50), and if this is acceptable, a larger pivotal study can be done. Lower-risk devices might progress to a pivotal study more quickly. Pivotal studies would be used to gain a marketing authorisation and need to be designed properly with both safety and efficacy outcomes. Specific considerations include:

- Clinical trials tend to have relatively few patients and not randomised, hence their evaluation could include high-quality real-world data
- They are rarely placebo-controlled because sham devices may be difficult to create or insert (especially if this requires an invasive procedure).
- For moderate or high risk devices all serious adverse events (SAEs) may need expedited reporting to the regulatory authorities (see section 'Safety monitoring and reporting' on page 185), whether the events are related to the device or not. This is in contrast to drug trials where only suspected unexpected serious adverse reactions (SUSARs, considered causally related to the drug) need to have expedited safety
- Patients may need to carry an implant card containing the device name, serial number and relevant warnings/precautions.
- Insertion of the device may require a specialist or surgeon, and there could be a learning curve for this as part of the trial.

Cell and gene therapy[22-25]

Cell and gene therapies are sometimes referred to as 'advanced therapies' or 'advanced therapy medicinal products' (ATMPs). They are considered to be high-risk treatments and are highly regulated. Clinical trials, therefore, have special scrutiny, requiring close safety monitoring of patients. They are often conducted in patients with advanced disorders who have already relapsed after standard therapies, and there are limited (if any) further treatment options.

Cell therapy involves taking a sample of a patient's cells, manipulating them in the laboratory (and in some cases modifying them genetically) before transferring them back to the patient with therapeutic intent. For cellular immunotherapy in oncology, the patient's own immune cells are modified, often to enable them to recognise and attack cancer cells. Most products are based on cells taken from the patient (autologous), but other products use cells from (matched) healthy donors (allogeneic) because they are easier to produce but there may be issues over rejection by the patient. Gene therapy aims to modify or manipulate the expression of an individual gene or correct abnormal genes in the patient's cells. Chimeric antigen receptor (CAR) T-cell therapy, is a major immunotherapy used for several cancer types and planned for other disorders.

Most advanced therapy trials have been single-arm studies involving relatively few patients (20–100), but randomised designs are increasingly used but unlikely to be blinded. Efficacy outcomes are similar to those used in trials of other interventions for the same disorder, although some advanced therapy trials are not sufficiently powered to evaluate relapse/progression and death rates, which might take too long. Specific biological endpoints include:

* persistence and duration of circulating cell products (e.g. CAR T cells) in the blood
* the ability to collect cells and manufacture enough product for the patient
* neurotoxicity and cytokine release syndrome (a form of systemic inflammatory response)
* graft-versus-host disease (GVHD) using allogeneic products
* a variety of biomarkers for response and toxicity, usually measured in blood.

These may include non-standard laboratory tests. Other outcome measures are details of adverse events, including number of hospitalisations, and time in hospital especially intensive care units if patients suffer a major side effect. Box 8.7 shows specific issues and challenges.

An example of a cell therapy trial (JULIET) is shown in Box 8.8.[26] It has the typical design features of many such trials: relatively small, single-arm and the primary outcome measure is a surrogate endpoint. It is designed like many other single-arm studies (see Figure 4.2, page 43). The efficacy results were excellent. The target response rate (used in the design and sample size) was 38%, but the trial achieved a higher effect (52%). Other outcomes (e.g. overall survival) also showed high efficacy for this poor prognosis patient group.

As part of the submission for HTA approval (NICE, England), the sponsor included an indirect comparison of overall survival due to the lack of a randomised control arm in the JULIET trial. However, the review panel had some issues which reflected general considerations by HTA reviewers when evaluating real-world data when used for indirect comparisons[27]:

* There were major baseline factor differences between the JULIET trial and the real-world observational study used by the sponsor.
* The comparator data came from a retrospective observational study of pixantrone monotherapy as salvage therapy, but this was rarely used in practice and has low efficacy.

Box 8.7 Some specific considerations for trials of advanced therapies

• Clinical trials of advanced therapies tend to be conducted in a few expert centres with access to highly specialised manufacturing

• Manufacturing cell therapy products is expensive and labour intensive, although more automated systems are being developed, and third-party 'universal' approaches are planned.

• There needs to be high quality manufacturing control standards and monitoring (even an apparently minor contamination could lead to suspension of production)

• In the event of product manufacturing failure, the protocol needs to have a clear and expedited pathway to other treatments for the patient.

• Sophisticated laboratory manufacturing processes need to be in place before the trial starts (e.g. receiving and storing cells, production and transport back to patients) to meet Good Manufacturing Practice (GMP) requirements (see Section 10.11, page 192).

• Production slots in the manufacturing laboratory could be limited by the time an eligible patient has been identified and consented to the study (so patients are treated with conventional therapies instead to avoid further delaying treatment).

• Multiple serial blood sampling is often required for efficacy and safety endpoints (sometimes bone marrow when feasible).

Box 8.8 Example of a trial of a cell therapy. Source: Schuster et al.[26]/figure reproduced with permission from the Massachusetts Medical Society/NEJM

Location: Multicentre in the US

Participants: Patients with diffuse large B-cell lymphoma who had relapsed after standard therapies

Intervention: CAR-T cell therapy tisagenlecleucel (anti-CD19)

Control: None, this was a single-arm clinical trial

Outcome measures: Overall tumour response rate (tumour had partially or completely regressed), and survival

Results: Response rate 52% (95% CI 41–62%). Overall survival:

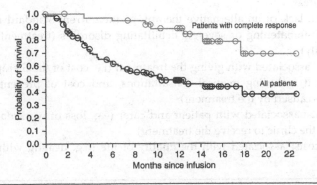

- NICE considered that *combination* chemotherapies are more commonly used as salvage (e.g. gemcitabine and oxaliplatin, with or without rituximab).
- Using data on combination chemotherapies made the comparison of survival between tisagenlecleucel and the control group less pronounced than the one submitted by the sponsor (illustrating that the choice of controls can influence comparative efficacy results)
- Although NICE had uncertainty over the magnitude of the overall survival benefit they approved the product, influenced by the high response rate from the clinical trial and that there is no standard treatment for this particular patient population (i.e. unmet need).

8.3 Health economic analyses[28-33]

In most societies, financial resources for healthcare are limited. With advances in medical treatments and an ageing population in many countries governments need to monitor how much to spend on public health and clinical services. Health economic evaluation is therefore an important consideration when investigating a new intervention, especially given the high cost of many new drugs. It essentially involves considering whether a new therapy represents 'value for money' and affordability by the healthcare service (Box 8.9). The term **financial toxicity** is used to describe situations where treatment costs are high and paid for by patients or their families, with an adverse impact on their personal finances and quality of life (stress, depression and anxiety). This is a particular issue in low and middle income countries.

Health economic evaluations tend to concentrate on the cost to the healthcare provider, because these cost items are easier to specify. It is also usual practice to standardise financial costs in the future to what they might be in present-day values allowing for inflation (called **discounting**). The effect of discounting is small when the costs and health benefits occur at the same time, but large when costs could be incurred over many years. Box 8.10 outlines four types of health economic analyses. Many trials now collect participant-level cost and resource-use data as part of the protocol and within the case report forms because this should produce a more comprehensive and reliable evaluation.

Box 8.9 General considerations about the costs of new interventions

- Cost of illness/burden of the disorder: the overall impact of the disorder on society
- Epidemiology of the disease: incidence/prevalence of the disorder, and in different geographical areas
- Unmet need: lack of an alternative therapy or the current standard of care has low efficacy, or life-threatening or severely debilitating disorders (treatment costs could be higher generally)
- Direct costs: associated with giving the treatment (i.e. cost of the therapy itself, cost of administering it including medical consultations, and cost of preventing or treating adverse effects caused by the treatment)
- Indirect costs: associated with patient and carer (e.g. loss of work days and income, travel costs to the clinic to receive the treatment)
- Intangible costs: associated with the quality of life (e.g. dealing with pain, physical immobility).

Box 8.10 Types of healthcare economic analyses informed by clinical trial data

---

- **Cost-effectiveness analysis:** a comparison of costs in monetary units with outcomes in quantitative non-monetary units (for example, reduced mortality or morbidity). The incremental cost-effectiveness ratio (ICER) is used.
- **E.g.** total cost of treating 200 people who had the New treatment is £30,000; and corresponding total cost of the control therapy is £20,000 for 200 people. The new treatment leads to 5 fewer events (e.g. deaths). ICER is 10,000/5=£4000 per life saved.
- **Cost–utility analysis:** a form of cost-effectiveness analysis that compares costs in monetary units with outcomes in terms of their utility, usually to the patient, measured in quality-adjusted life years QALY). The cost per QALY gained is used.
- E.g. $Cost_{new}$ and $Cost_{control}$ are for example the mean cost in each group. Each participant has a QoL profile over time and hence an area under the curve.

$$Ratio = \frac{cost_{new} - cost_{control}}{Mean\_Area_{new} - Mean\_Area_{control}} = \frac{£25,000 - £10,000}{3.2 - 1.5} = \frac{£15,000}{1.7} = £8823$$

£8,823, is the cost per one QALY gained (i.e. the marginal cost), i.e. how much it costs to gain an extra year of healthy life using the new intervention.

- **Cost-minimisation analysis:** determining the cheapest therapy when they have similar efficacy (evidence from non-inferiority or equivalence trials)
- **Cost–benefit analysis:** a comparison of costs and benefits, both of which are quantified in common monetary terms, and can include a person's willingness to pay for the expected benefit associated with a new therapy, to be compared with the direct cost of the therapy.

References

1. Toumi M. *Introduction to Market Access for Pharmaceuticals*. CRC Press, 2017.
2. Venter WDF, Moorhouse M, Sokhela S *et al*. Dolutegravir plus two different prodrugs of Tenofovir to treat HIV. *N Engl J Med* 2019; **381**(9):803–815.
3. IQWiG Reports – Commission No. A13-20. Ocriplasmin for the treatment of vitreomacular traction (VMT) in adults. `https://www.iqwig.de/download/a13-20_ocriplasmin_extract-of-dossier-assessment.pdf`.
4. FDA review of erdafitinib for treating metastatic urothelial carcinoma. NDA/BLA Multi-disciplinary Review and Evaluation (NDA [NME] 212018). `https://www.accessdata.fda.gov/drugsat-fda_docs/nda/2019/212018Orig1s000MultidisciplineR.pdf`.
5. Feinberg BA, Gajra A, Zettler ME *et al*. Use of real-world evidence to support FDA approval of oncology drugs. *Value Health* 2020; **23**(10):1358–1365.
6. McCulloch P, Cook JA, Altman DG *et al*. IDEAL framework for surgical innovation 1: the idea and development stages. *BMJ* 2013; **346**:f3012.
7. Ergina PL, Barkun JS, McCulloch P *et al*.; IDEAL Group. IDEAL framework for surgical innovation 2: observational studies in the exploration and assessment stages. BMJ 2013; **346**:f3011.
8. Cook JA, McCulloch P, Blazeby JM *et al*. IDEAL framework for surgical innovation 3: randomised controlled trials in the assessment stage and evaluations in the long term study stage. *BMJ* 2013; **346**:f2820.
9. Moseley JB, O'Malley K, Petersen NJ *et al*. A controlled trial of arthroscopic surgery for osteoarthritis of the knee. *N Engl J Med* 2002; **347**(2):81–88.

10. Deprest JA, Nicolaides KH, Benachi A *et al.*; TOTAL Trial for Severe Hypoplasia Investigators. Randomized trial of fetal surgery for severe left diaphragmatic hernia. *N Engl J Med* 2021; **385**(2):107–118.

11. Deprest JA, Benachi A, Gratacos E *et al.*; TOTAL Trial for Moderate Hypoplasia Investigators. Randomized trial of fetal surgery for moderate left diaphragmatic hernia. N Engl J Med 2021; **385**(2):119–129.

12. Ramirez PT, Frumovitz M, Pareja R *et al.* Minimally invasive versus abdominal radical hysterectomy for cervical cancer. *N Engl J Med* 2018; **379**(20):1895–1904.

13. Rangan A, Handoll H, Brealey S, et al; PROFHER trial collaborators. surgical vs nonsurgical treatment of adults with displaced fractures of the proximal humerus: the PROFHER randomized clinical trial JAMA 2015; 313(10):1037–47

14. Thompson MK, Poortmans P, Chalmers AJ *et al.* Practice-changing radiation therapy trials for the treatment of cancer: where are we 150 years after the birth of Marie Curie? *Br J Cancer* 2018; **119**:389–407.

15. Sharma RA, Plummer R, Stock JK *et al.* Clinical development of new drug-radiotherapy combinations. *Nat Rev Clin Oncol* 2016; 13:627–642.

16. Edmond SN, Turk DC, Williams DA, Kerns RD. Considerations of trial design and conduct in behavioral interventions for the management of chronic pain in adults. *Pain Rep* 2018; **4**(3):e65.

17. Younge JO, Kouwenhoven-Pasmooij TA, Freak-Poli R *et al.* Randomized study designs for lifestyle interventions: a tutorial. *Int J Epidemiol* 2015; **44**(6):2006–2019.

18. Delgado-Lista J, Alcala-Diaz JF, Torres-Peña JD *et al.*; CORDIOPREV Investigators. Long-term secondary prevention of cardiovascular disease with a Mediterranean diet and a low-fat diet (CORDIOPREV): a randomised controlled trial. *Lancet* 2022; **399**(10338):1876–1885.

19. Faris O, Shuren J. An FDA viewpoint on unique considerations for medical-device clinical trials. *N Engl J Med* 2017; **376**(14):1350–1357.

20. Resnic FS, Matheny ME. Medical devices in the real world. *N Engl J Med* 2018; **378**(7):595–597.

21. Neugebauer EAM, Rath A, Antoine SL *et al.* Specific barriers to the conduct of randomised clinical trials on medical devices. *Trials* 2017; **18**(1):427.

22. Exley AR, Rantell K, McBlane J. Clinical development of cell therapies for cancer: the regulators' perspective. *Eur J Cancer* 2020; **138**:41–53.

23. FDA guidance on trials of gene and cell therapies. `https://www.fda.gov/regulatory-information/search-fda-guidance-documents/considerations-design-early-phase-clinical-trials-cellular-and-gene-therapy-products`.

24. Abou-El-Enein M, Hey SP. Cell and gene therapy trials: are we facing an 'evidence crisis'? *eClinicalMedicine* 2019; **7**:13–14.

25. Ginn SL, Amaya AK, Alexander IE, Edelstein M, Abedi MR. Gene therapy clinical trials worldwide to 2017: an update. *J Gene Med* 2018; 20:e3015.

26. Schuster SJ, Bishop MR, Tam CS *et al.*; JULIET Investigators. Tisagenlecleucel in adult relapsed or refractory diffuse large B-cell lymphoma. *Engl J Med* 2019; **380**(1):45–56.

27. `https://www.nice.org.uk/guidance/ta567/resources/tisagenlecleucel-for-treating-relapsed-or-refractory-diffuse-large-bcell-lymphoma-after-2-or-more-systemic-therapies-pdf-82607087377861`.

28. Glick HA, Doshi JA, Sonnad SS, Polsky D. *Economic Evaluation in Clinical Trials*. 2nd edn, Oxford University Press, 2014.

29. Raftery J. Economic evaluation: an introduction. *BMJ* 1998; **316**:1013–1014.

30. Raftery J. Costing in economic evaluation. *BMJ* 2000; **320**:1597.

31. Robinson R. Economic evaluation and health care: what does it mean? *BMJ* 1993; **307**:670–673.

32. van Boven JFM, van de Hei SJ, Sadatsafavi M. Making sense of cost-effectiveness analyses in respiratory medicine: a practical guide for non-health economists. *Eur Respir J* 2019; **53**(3):1801816.

33. Sanders GD, Maciejewski ML, Basu A. Overview of cost-effectiveness analysis. *JAMA* 2019; **321**(14):1400–1401.

CHAPTER 9

Systematic reviews and meta-analyses; and real-world evidence

Previous chapters presented key features of the design, analysis and interpretation of a single clinical trial. However, it is possible to combine information (e.g. efficacy or adverse events) from several studies; Figure 9.1.This can be done using only randomised studies based on direct comparisons (Section 9.1), or by comparing two or more interventions where participants were not randomly allocated to them (indirect comparisons). Indirect comparisons could be based on randomised studies only (Section 9.2) or a combination of clinical trials and real-world data/observational studies (Section 9.3); Figure 9.1. They can be particularly useful as supporting evidence for a randomised trial or where a randomised study is not feasible. However, the limitations of the design and analysis features of indirect comparisons and real-world data mean that some decision-makers (e.g. health technology assessment agencies) do not always accept this type of evidence.

9.1 Systematic reviews of randomised controlled trials (direct comparisons)

Systematic reviews are usually not the same as review articles, which may be presented as narratives based on selected papers. They may therefore reflect the personal and professional interests of the author and be biased towards the positive (or negative) studies. Such reviews tend to describe the features of each paper without trying to combine the quantitative results. The assessment of several trials together needs to be done in a **systematic** and unbiased way. Systematic reviews tend to be conducted on randomised phase II or III trials, but they can also be done for single-arm trials (Box 9.1).[1-9]

Sources of published systematic reviews
The Cochrane Collaboration is a well-known collection of systematic reviews that are available on their website. There are established Collaborative Review Groups who undertake systematic reviews to a similar standard, and sometimes updated regularly:
- Cochrane Collaboration (`http://www.cochrane.org`)
- The Cochrane Library (`http://www3.interscience.wiley.com/cgi-bin/mrwhome/106568753/HOME`)

This website also has an online guide on how to conduct and analysis reviews: `https://training.cochrane.org/handbook/current`.

A Concise Guide to Clinical Trials, Second Edition. Allan Hackshaw.
© 2024 John Wiley & Sons Ltd. Published 2024 by John Wiley & Sons Ltd.

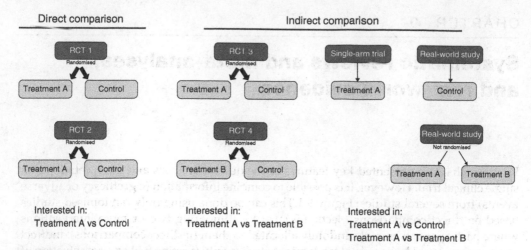

Figure 9.1 Examples of different ways of combining information from several studies. RCT, randomised controlled trial.

Box 9.1 Main purposes of a systematic review and meta-analysis

To confirm existing practice but provide a more precise estimate of the treatment effect

- The combined effect size should have greater precision (narrower 95%CI), and the result is more likely to be statistically significant than individual trials.
- It is possible to detect smaller treatment effects.
- Subgroup analyses may be more reliable because they have more participants or events.

To change existing practice

- Some systematic reviews have led to a new intervention being adopted into practice, but usually they have resulted in an existing treatment becoming more commonly used.
- Reviews are often used to develop national guidelines for defining standard practice.

To determine whether new trials are needed

- A systematic review can show that there are only a few small published trials, perhaps with inconsistent results.
- Taken together, they provide insufficient evidence for a treatment; hence, a large new trial is justified.

Stages of a systematic review

Health professionals need to keep abreast of new developments, and systematic reviews are valuable summaries of the evidence. A systematic review is a research project in its own right that can be a lengthy undertaking, but it is only as good as the studies on which it is based. A review of mainly small, poorly designed trials can be inferior to a single large, well-designed trial. An example of this is the evaluation of dietary supplementation with enteral lactoferrin (a natural antibiotic protein from cow's milk) for very preterm infants to prevent late-onset infection. A review of 6 RCTs showed a strong risk reduction (pooled relative risk 0.59, 95%CI 0.40-0.87), but they had variable design qualities, with

---

Box 9.2 Stages of a systematic review

1. Define the research question, and identify the appropriate outcome measures.
2. Specify a list of criteria for including and excluding studies.
3. Undertake a literature search using electronic databases (e.g. PubMed, Medline and Embase) and after reading the abstracts identify articles that might be appropriate.
4. Obtain the full papers identified from the literature search. The reference lists of these papers are also used to identify additional papers not found in the electronic search.
5. Apply the inclusion criteria to produce the final list of trials to be analysed.
6. Critically appraise each report and extract specific relevant information. Alternatively, request the raw participant-level data from the trial investigators, as part of a joint collaborative project.
7. Perform a **meta-analysis** to combine the individual effect sizes into a single estimate.
8. Interpret and summarise the findings, including limitations of the review.

---

study size ranging from only 47 to 321 infants.[10] However, a single large RCT of 2203 infants showed no benefit (relative risk 0.95).[11]

The systematic review process is outlined in Box 9.2.[12] The summary data (i.e. effect sizes) and participant baseline characteristics are extracted from the published papers. Alternatively, the raw data are requested from the authors, called an **individual patient/ participant data (IPD) meta-analysis**, and once they are sent to a central depository (after being collected, collated and checked), there is essentially a single large data set.

Meta-analysis

The main stage of a systematic review is combining the effect sizes into a single estimate using a statistical technique called **meta-analysis**. Several methods are available, and they essentially obtain an average of the effect size weighted by the standard error to avoid small unreliable studies having equal importance as large studies.[12]

Figure 9.2 is a typical meta-analysis plot (a **forest plot**), associated with a review of nicotine replacement therapy (NRT).[13] The software RevMan can be used.[14] It shows the individual results from 13 randomised trials of self-referred smokers who were randomised to receive either 2 mg nicotine chewing gum or control (such as placebo gum). The main outcome measure is the proportion of smokers who had stopped smoking one year after starting treatment, and the effect size is the ratio of these proportions (i.e. risk ratio or relative risk). The studies are ordered by the magnitude of the effect size but this can also be done by year of publication. Forest plots can be derived for any type of effect size.

The **weight** given to each trial is calculated from the **standard error** (measure of precision, Figure 6.8, page 95) of the risk ratio, on a logarithmic scale.

Weight is a measure of the relative importance of an individual trial in a review

Weight $= 1/\text{standard error}^2$

Studies with small standard errors (e.g. many participants/events) have large weights

Studies with large standard errors (e.g. few participants/events) have small weights

---

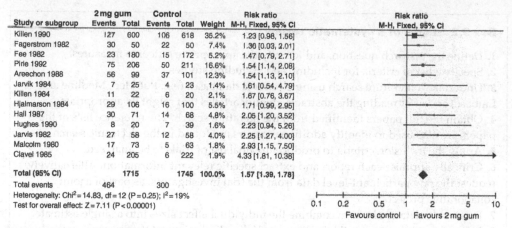

Study or subgroup	2 mg gum Events	2 mg gum Total	Control Events	Control Total	Weight	Risk ratio M-H, Fixed, 95% CI
Killen 1990	127	600	106	618	35.2%	1.23 [0.98, 1.56]
Fagerstrom 1982	30	50	22	50	7.4%	1.36 [0.03, 2.01]
Fee 1982	23	180	15	172	5.2%	1.47 [0.79, 2.71]
Pirie 1992	75	206	50	211	16.6%	1.54 [1.14, 2.08]
Areechon 1988	56	99	37	101	12.3%	1.54 [1.13, 2.10]
Jarvik 1984	7	25	4	23	1.4%	1.61 [0.54, 4.79]
Killen 1984	11	22	6	20	2.1%	1.67 [0.76, 3.67]
Hjalmarson 1984	29	106	16	100	5.5%	1.71 [0.99, 2.95]
Hall 1987	30	71	14	68	4.8%	2.05 [1.20, 3.52]
Hughes 1990	8	20	7	39	1.6%	2.23 [0.94, 5.26]
Jarvis 1982	27	58	12	58	4.0%	2.25 [1.27, 4.00]
Malcolm 1980	17	73	5	63	1.8%	2.93 [1.15, 7.50]
Clavel 1985	24	205	6	222	1.9%	4.33 [1.81, 10.38]
Total (95% CI)		1715		1745	100.0%	1.57 [1.39, 1.78]
Total events	464		300			

Heterogeneity: Chi² = 14.83, df = 12 (P = 0.25); I² = 19%
Test for overall effect: Z = 7.11 (P < 0.00001)

Figure 9.2 Example of a forest plot from a meta-analysis of randomised trials evaluating nicotine replacement therapy (2 mg nicotine chewing gum) for smoking cessation. The figure was created using the published results from *Tang et al.*[13] and RevMan.[14] CI: confidence interval; M-H Mantel-Haenszel method, which can handle trials with few participants or few events. The no-effect value is 1.0. If the 95% CI excludes one, the result is statistically significant.

In Figure 9.2, each weight is expressed as a percentage of the sum of all the weights across trials, allowing a comparison of the relative contribution that each trial makes to the analysis. The size of the central square for each trial is proportional to the weight, so that greater visual attention is made to the most reliable (e.g. largest) studies.

Weight (standard error) is most influenced by the number of events (here, the number of people who stopped smoking):

• Killen 1990 has the largest weight (35.2%) because it has *both* a large number of participants (600 + 618) and events (127 + 106).
• Clavel 1985 has a small weight (1.9%) because it has few events (24 + 6) despite being a fairly large trial (205 + 222).
• Areechon 1988 has a moderate weight (12.3%) because it has many events (56 + 37) even though it is not a particularly large trial (99 + 101).

The statistical techniques used in a meta-analysis allow for the weight of each trial when combining the effect sizes. Examples of methods are Mantel-Haenszel, Peto odds ratio, Peto's 'observed-expected number of events' statistic and Dersimonian and Laird. Other approaches ('exact methods') can handle rare events. The simplest general method is shown in Box 9.3.

In Figure 9.2, the pooled risk ratio is 1.57 with 95%CI 1.39–1.78. These are interpreted in the same way as if they came from a single trial. Smokers who used nicotine gum

---

Box 9.3 Estimating the combined effect size (fixed effects model)

$$\text{Combined effect size} = \frac{\text{sum of}\left(\text{effect size} \times \text{weight for each trial}\right)}{\text{sum of all the weights}}$$

The effect size could be a mean difference, absolute risk difference, relative risk or hazard ratio (the latter two are used on a $\log_e$ scale, and the result is anti-logged).

were 57% more likely to quit than the controls. Note that the CI is narrower than any individual trial, and the p-value is very small (Test for overall effect $p < 0.00001$) – which is what meta-analyses aim to achieve.

Heterogeneity

No two trials are identical. There are two forms of **heterogeneity**: (i) differences in design and conduct which are examined qualitatively, and (ii) differences between the effect sizes which can be quantified (hereafter called statistical heterogeneity). If either form of heterogeneity is present and substantial, combining the results into a single estimate may be inappropriate.

There are two statistical tests for heterogeneity associated with the effect sizes (Figure 9.2)[12,15]:

- The test for heterogeneity compares how different the individual effect sizes are from the combined value, and whether observed differences are compatible with chance alone assuming that there is a single underlying true effect. Here, the p-value is 0.25; hence, there is insufficient evidence of heterogeneity using this approach. The 'test for heterogeneity' may lack statistical power when there are few trials or they have few participants.
- I^2 reflects the percentage of variability in effect sizes across the trial that is due to real differences and not chance ($I^2 = 0\%$ indicates no heterogeneity at all, and $I^2 = 100\%$ indicates considerable heterogeneity). Here $I^2 = 19\%$, which again does not indicate much heterogeneity. This measure is more robust when there are few trials.

Roughly, $I^2 =$

0–30%: acceptably low heterogeneity

30–60%: moderate heterogeneity

60–90%: substantial heterogeneity

90–100%: considerable heterogeneity.

Fixed or random effects model to combine the results

There are two common approaches to obtaining a weighted average of the effect sizes, and the choice is often influenced by the presence of heterogeneity between the effect sizes:

- A **fixed effects model**, indicated by the word 'Fixed' at the top right-hand side of Figure 9.2, assumes that there is a single underlying treatment effect. This method provides the best estimate of the true treatment effect. It can be relatively simple (Box 9.3).
- A **random effects model** ('Random' appears in the forest plot) assumes that the trials are estimating different but related treatment effects. A common method is by DerSimonian and Laird,[16] and it incorporates the extent of heterogeneity (variability) between the effect sizes. This method provides an estimate of the average treatment effect.

The two models produce almost the same pooled result if there is no statistical heterogeneity. When there is significant heterogeneity, they can produce quite different results,

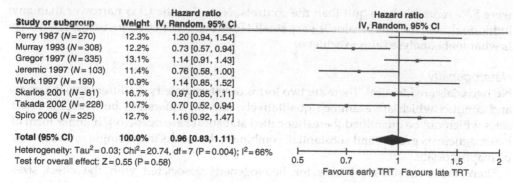

Study or subgroup	Weight	Hazard ratio IV, Random, 95% CI
Perry 1987 ($N = 270$)	12.3%	1.20 [0.94, 1.54]
Murray 1993 ($N = 308$)	12.2%	0.73 [0.57, 0.94]
Gregor 1997 ($N = 335$)	13.1%	1.14 [0.91, 1.43]
Jeremic 1997 ($N = 103$)	11.4%	0.76 [0.58, 1.00]
Work 1997 ($N = 199$)	10.9%	1.14 [0.85, 1.52]
Skarlos 2001 ($N = 81$)	16.7%	0.97 [0.85, 1.11]
Takada 2002 ($N = 228$)	10.7%	0.70 [0.52, 0.94]
Spiro 2006 ($N = 325$)	12.7%	1.16 [0.92, 1.47]
Total (95% CI)	**100.0%**	**0.96 [0.83, 1.11]**

Heterogeneity: Tau^2 = 0.03; Chi^2 = 20.74, df = 7 (P = 0.004); I^2 = 66%
Test for overall effect: Z = 0.55 (P = 0.58)

Favours early TRT   Favours late TRT

Figure 9.3 Forest plot of eight randomised trials comparing the timing of thoracic radiotherapy (TRT); i.e. given when standard chemotherapy starts ('early TRT') or at the end of chemotherapy ('late TRT'), in patients with small-cell lung cancer. The primary endpoint is overall survival, and the trials are ordered by year of publication. The figure was created using the published results from *Spiro et al* and RevMan.[14,17]

and the random effects approach leads to a wider 95%CI. If a random effects model were used for the smoking cessation trial, the combined risk ratio would become 1.61, 95%CI 1.38–1.86. This is sufficiently close to 1.57 (the difference reflects the small amount of heterogeneity), and a slightly wider 95%CI is observed.

A random effects model is often used when heterogeneity is considered to be present. While it attempts to incorporate *statistical* heterogeneity, it does not account for/adjust for qualitative heterogeneity (differences in design and conduct).

Figure 9.3 is an example of a meta-analysis of eight trials evaluating whether giving thoracic radiotherapy early is more effective than giving it later, among patients with lung cancer.[17] The effect sizes are clearly very different. Both the test for heterogeneity ($p = 0.004$) and I^2 (66%) indicate significant heterogeneity. A random effects model *seems* appropriate, which produces a hazard ratio of 0.96 ($p = 0.58$), suggesting no effect of early TRT (reflecting the average treatment effect).

However, it is essential to investigate the possible causes of heterogeneity from the individual trial papers, which requires knowledge about the disease area and type of interventions. In Figure 9.3, two trials (Murray 1993 and Spiro 2006) had practically the same design and protocol, yet one showed a clear benefit for early TRT and the other did not. This discordance led to an in-depth appraisal of all trials which identified the most likely reason for the heterogeneity: the delivery of the standard (background) chemotherapy (Table 9.1). The appropriate conclusion was that early TRT is beneficial, but only if the background chemotherapy can be completed. The pooled effect from all eight trials is inappropriate, and using the random effects model does not fix the underlying heterogeneity, and would yield an incorrect conclusion. There are essentially two separate meta-analyses.

Considerations when evaluating a systematic review

There are several aspects to consider when deciding whether a systematic review provides good evidence for or against a new intervention (Box 9.4). **Publication bias** can be an important issue, and a funnel plot (Figure 9.4) can be used to see if there is a potential problem with under-reported studies.[5,18]

Table 9.1 Investigation of heterogeneity in the meta-analysis in Figure 9.3.

Trials (first author)	Standard chemotherapy:	Individual hazard ratios and I^2	Combined hazard ratio (95%CI)
Murray, Jeremic, Takada	High adherence *and similar* between the TRT trial arms	0.73, 0.76, 0.70 $I^2 = 0\%$	0.73 (0.62–0.86) $p < 0.001$ Early TRT beneficial
Perry, Gregor, Work, Skarlos, Spiro	Lower adherence in the early TRT trial arm	1.20, 1.14, 1.14, 0.97, 1.16 $I^2 = 0\%$	1.07 (0.98–1.17) $p = 0.15$ No effect of early TRT
All trials		$I^2 = 66\%$	0.96 (0.83–1.11) $p = 0.58$ No effect of early TRT

TRT: thoracic radiotherapy.

Box 9.4 Key considerations when evaluating a systematic review

Item	Comments
Identification and selection of trials	A thorough literature search, including the references within papers, should yield most/all studies. Carefully considered search terms are essential.* The aim is to show that many trials have not been missed.
Participants	This should be *broadly similar* between the trials. An intervention can have differential effects between, e.g. low- and high-risk populations; hence, combining these may not be appropriate or meaningful.
Definitions of the interventions and outcome measures	These would not be identical between the trials but, as above, need to be *broadly comparable*. The results can be particularly sensitive to very different definitions of endpoints.
Heterogeneity	This is often not well addressed. If there is clear heterogeneity between the effect sizes a thorough examination of the design and conduct features is warranted, though this still may not provide the likely cause(s).
Publication bias[5,18]	Trials with negative results (small or no treatment benefit) may be less likely to be published, so the combined effect size from the meta-analysis might be overestimated.
Study quality	This can be evaluated using various criteria for meta-analyses, applied to the trial design, conduct or analysis. These often categorise each item as having a 'low' or 'high' risk of bias. This is a subjective exercise that could produce a biased selection of studies to be used in the analysis. It is perhaps best to include all trials and then exclude those considered 'poor quality' to see how the results compare.

*Including being aware of differences in spelling (e.g. 'tumor' in the US and 'tumour' in Europe).

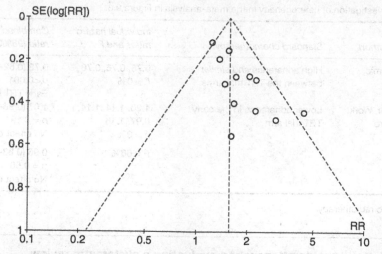

Figure 9.4 Funnel plot for the 13 smoking cessation trials in Figure 9.2. The effect size RR (relative risk) on the x-axis is plotted against the weight (1/standard error, or standard error) on the y-axis. If the spread of the observations within the triangle is asymmetric, this is evidence of possible publication bias. Figure created using the studies in Tang *et al* and RevMan.[13, 14]. Although there is a hint of this the number of trials is insufficient to tell for sure. [There are two overlapping circles for RR 1.54.]

Reporting systematic reviews

There are standard guidelines for reporting and publishing systematic reviews.[19, 20] They must include:

- The detailed search strategy, search terms, and databases were used.
- The eligibility criteria for inclusion in the meta-analysis.
- Specifying the total number of abstracts found during the electronic search, how many full articles were examined, how many were used in the meta-analysis, how many were excluded and the reasons for their exclusion.
- A table summarising the main characteristics of each trial used in the meta-analysis, such as geographical location, time period when the trial was conducted, sample size, population (e.g. age range and gender distribution), the interventions and the effect size.
- Method of statistical analysis (fixed or random effects model), the effect size used, and any investigation of heterogeneity if it exists, such as a formal statistical test or I^2 value.
- Interpretation of the results, and their implication for clinical practice.

9.2 Meta-analyses based on indirect comparisons

The meta-analyses outlined in Section 9.1 were based on an intervention that was directly compared with a similar control therapy across several RCTs. There are now several standards of care for many disorders making it difficult for trials of new therapies to always compare them with the same control group. Furthermore, pharmaceutical companies, for example, may be reluctant to directly compare their drug with a competitor's (referred to as **head-to-head comparisons**, particularly when the drugs are in the same biological class). Nevertheless, there is interest in knowing how well different therapies compare (efficacy or safety) even if they had not been evaluated in the same trial.

Indirect comparisons (specifically called **mixed treatment comparisons** or **network meta-analyses**) involve estimating an effect size between two interventions that were not directly compared in an RCT trial. Figure 9.5 shows the basic premise. The simple statistical approach in the figure can rarely be used due to differences in the trial designs. Sophisticated statistical methods (e.g. Bayesian statistics) are used instead. Box 9.5 outlines the main concepts.

An example of a network meta-analysis is shown in Figure 9.6, that evaluated several EGFR inhibitors for treating advanced lung cancer where the tumour is EGFR-positive.[21] Connecting lines indicate trials that have directly compared two treatments in an RCT: more trials are reflected by a thicker line. The size of each solid circle reflects the number of patients given the treatment (also shown in brackets). Relatively few RCTs have directly compared the EGFR inhibitors.

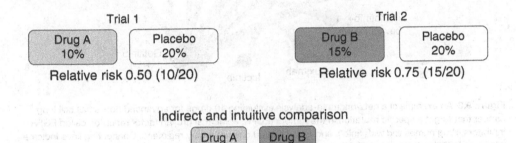

Relative risk 0.67 (0.50/0.75)

This is OK if trials are *very* similar

Figure 9.5 Illustration of the concept of an indirect comparison.

Box 9.5 Outline of the general approach to indirect comparison meta-analyses

- Statistical methods (e.g. Bayesian) are more complex than meta-analyses of RCTs that compare a similar experimental therapy with a similar control therapy.
- Uses information from the direct comparison RCTs (e.g. measures of variability and heterogeneity) to estimate treatment effects:
   - between two therapies that had been directly compared in an RCT
   - between two therapies that had no direct RCT
- Uses statistical modelling/regression methods (frequentist or Bayesian):
   - Frequentist models: use the observed data*
   - Bayesian models: assume and incorporate 'prior' numerical estimates of e.g. heterogeneity from other data sources
- Produces a grid of effect sizes and 95%CIs for all possible treatment pairs

RCT: randomised controlled trial.

* As with the examples in Section 9.1.

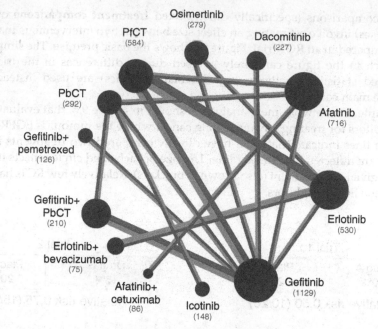

Figure 9.6 An example of a network meta-analysis evaluating 10 drugs for advanced non-small cell lung cancer that target a specific mutation in the tumour (EGFR, epidermal growth factor receptor, called EGFR inhibitors, drug names end with 'inib'), and two standard chemotherapy regimens. Connecting lines indicate where an RCT has been done. PbCT, pemetrexed-based chemotherapy; PfCT, pemetrexed-free chemotherapy. Source: Zhao et al.[21]/figure reproduced with permission from the BMJ.

Box 9.6 shows selected comparisons from the treatments shown in Figure 9.6, in a typical grid format.[21] The analyses (modelling) provide effect sizes for all possible pairs of treatment comparisons. The grid often shows two outcome measures (here, PFS and OS).

- Hazard ratio (HR) for PFS for osimertinib versus erlotinib is 0.48; the risk (hazard) of progressing or dying is halved in patients who had osimertinib (which is statistically significant because the 95% credible interval excludes the no effect value 1).
- HR for OS for erlotinib versus osimertinib is 1.59; the risk (hazard) of dying is *increased* in patients who had erlotinib (statistically significant). This can easily be switched to osimertinib versus erlotinib by taking the reciprocal: 0.63 (1/1.59), and the direction of effect is now the same as for PFS.
- There is no trial directly comparing osimertinib and dacomitinib (no connecting line in Figure 9.6) but the analyses produce an effect size for them: PFS HR 0.74 for osimertinib versus dacomitinib, and OS HR 1.21 for dacomitinib versus osimertinib (which becomes 0.83 [1/1.21] for osimertinib versus dacomitinib).

The analyses can also produce Bayesian ranking profiles for each of the 12 interventions shown in Figure 9.6. A ranking plot for osimertinib is shown in Figure 9.7. This therapy is most likely to be ranked first (i.e. has the greatest efficacy/benefit) for PFS out of all 12 therapies (cumulative probability 57%), and ~28% probability of being ranked first for OS.

Box 9.6 Estimates of hazard ratios (95% credible intervals)* for overall and progression-free survival for selected treatment comparisons in Figure 9.6. The ordering of the comparison for each hazard ratio is row treatment by column treatment. Effect sizes in bold reflect statistical significance

		Progression-free survival (PFS)		
Overall survival (OS)	Osimertinib	**0.74 (0.55–1.00)**	**0.52 (0.40–0.68)**	**0.48 (0.40–0.57)**
	1.21 (0.83–1.76)	Dacomitinib	0.70 (0.52-0.95)	0.65 (0.48-0.87)
	1.32 (0.97–1.80)	1.10 (0.79–1.54)	Afatinib	0.92 (0.72-1.18)
	1.59 (1.23–2.06)	1.33 (0.94–1.87)	1.21 (0.93–1.55)	Erlotinib

*Credible intervals are produced by Bayesian methods instead of confidence intervals, but they can be thought of as having a broadly similar interpretation (i.e. measure of precision).

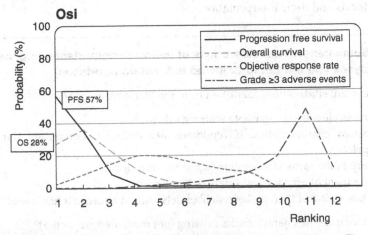

Figure 9.7 Bayesian ranking profile plot for osimertinib from the network meta-analyses in Figure 9.6, in which there are 12 treatments (hence 12 possible ranks). The y-axis is the (cumulative) probability for osimertinib to have each rank (x-axis) for the different endpoints. The probabilities of osimertinib being ranked first (for PFS or OS) are shown: 57% and 28%. Source: Zhao et al.[21]/figure reproduced with permission from the BMJ.

Several statistical checks can be performed, including:

- **Heterogeneity** in the original effect sizes between trials that had the same direct comparisons (similar principle as in Section 9.1). As before, the statistical methods do not account for qualitative heterogeneity between the studies.
- **Inconsistency**: the analyses (modelling) can produce a combined effect size based on studies that had a direct comparison of Treatments A and B, but also an estimate assuming A and B were indirect comparisons. These two effect sizes should be

comparable if the modelling is generally reliable. For example, in Figure 9.6, a few trials directly compared osimertinib and erlotinib. Using PFS, the direct effect was 0.78, and the indirect effect was 0.64 ($p = 0.47$). With numerous treatments, there is likely to be one or more comparisons where this consistency check may not appear favourable by chance.

Matching-adjusted indirect comparison (MAIC) is another approach that involves combining information from different sources, often for evaluating a single intervention. It involves using *raw (individual) participant data* from a clinical trial of one intervention (could be a single-arm or randomised trial) and *summary data* from another trial of another intervention usually taken from a journal article. This could be a new treatment versus control therapy, or a head-to-head comparison of two standards of care. Because the participant baseline characteristics are expected to be different between the different trials (randomisation was not used), the method uses propensity scores (covered in Section 9.3) to create a dataset from the trial with raw (participant-level) data that has similar baseline characteristics to the trial for which only summary data are available. An effect size is calculated if this is achieved.

Methods for indirect comparisons use complex and sophisticated statistical techniques. They can provide potentially useful evidence for comparing two or more interventions in the absence of direct comparison clinical trials. Box 9.7 lists some general considerations of these methods and their interpretation.

Box 9.7 Some general considerations of indirect comparisons (e.g. network meta-analyses and matching-adjusted indirect comparisons)

Have all relevant studies been identified from the literature search?

Whether the studies are comparable with regards to:
- Participant characteristics: if fundamentally different, combining data may be inappropriate.*
- Delivery of the same intervention (e.g. dose, duration).
- Measurement of efficacy and safety outcomes.
- Also, has a control therapy been deliberately chosen because it has low efficacy?

Are important baseline characteristics missing (not measured/reported)?

Is there significant heterogeneity in the quantitative effects?

Statistical methods:
- More complex than standard meta-analyses (Section 9.1), many use Bayesian methods and specialist software.
- Different methods have different assumptions and modelling approaches.
- Investigators should perform sensitivity analyses (i.e. try out different methods and assumptions to see how consistent the results are).
- Confounding and bias may still not be sufficiently dealt with, so the results are unreliable.

*E.g. if one trial only has high-risk participants and another trial only has low-risk participants, a treatment may not have the same effect in both.

9.3 Real-world evidence and real-world data

RCTs are the most reliable way to assess the efficacy and safety of a new intervention.[22] However, they can be difficult to do, especially for rare disorders, and for precision medicine where biomarkers are used to define small subgroups of people with the same marker (e.g. genetic mutation, or gene expression) who have or will develop a disorder. **Real-world data (RWD)** and **real-world evidence (RWE)** are meant to fill an evidence gap when RCTs are not feasible, or they provide supporting evidence for pivotal (e.g. phase III) randomised studies.

There are various definitions of RWD and RWE, and the following may be a helpful distinction:[23–26]

- RWD: the raw participant-level data collected from a study or electronic health records based on participants seen in real-life clinical care
- RWE: the analysis, synthesis and interpretation of RWD from one or more data source

---

RWE can include 'pragmatic' randomised trials conducted in routine practice, where eligibility, the interventions (random allocation, then administration), and assessment of efficacy and safety can be largely done using medical records with minimal contact and clinic visits. However, the majority of RWD comes from observational studies, which is the focus of this section. Potential limitations of randomised trials are meant to be addressed by RWD; Box 9.8. Figure 9.8 indicates typical uses of RWD. Four common ones are to compare:

- outcomes from the new treatment arm of an RCT (efficacy) with those from people given the new therapy in routine practice (RWD, effectiveness).
- a standard therapy (RWD) with other standard therapies (RWD).
- a new therapy (RCT) with several other standard treatments (RWD) as indirect comparisons.
- an unlicensed therapy (single-arm clinical trial) with a standard/licensed therapy (RWD) as the comparator. This might be the only realistic option for uncommon disorders.

Although RWD can provide supporting evidence for randomised trials, the limitations of RWD always need to be considered: lack of randomisation could lead to confounding and bias; unmeasured confounding; missing data; lower study/data quality; and methodological issues with the analyses. Any of these could contribute to unreliable results. Furthermore, RWD should not be a substitute for a well-designed RCT where such studies are feasible.

In addition to examining effectiveness, RWD can be used to monitor adverse events (pharmacoepidemiology), or examine adherence and find ways to improve this if it is too low.

Box 9.9 lists the types and sources of RWD. The concept of 'big data' is often applied to RWD because it involves the synthesis and analysis of large amounts of data collected electronically: **electronic health records (EHR)**.

When evaluating the benefits of an intervention, the term **efficacy** is often applied to randomised trials, and **effectiveness** to RWD.# Efficacy is analogous to testing the

---

\# These are not universal definitions, and some people consider them to be the same thing.

> **Box 9.8 Some general possible limitations of randomised controlled trials (RCT), and potential strengths of real-world evidence (RWE)**
>
> **RCTs – limitations**
>
> - Unrepresentative of the target or intended-use population, e.g. not enough women, ethnic minorities, lower socioeconomic groups, elderly or those with co-morbidities
> - Difficult choosing a single control/comparator therapy when there are several standards of care
> - Conducted in expert centres (e.g. might contribute to better efficacy, especially in unblinded trials)
> - Can require many assessments (e.g. clinic visits, scans, blood tests) which can put off patients/public and health professionals
> - Low accrual or long duration
> - Burdensome and expensive processes to set up and conduct trials
>
> **RWE – strengths**
>
> - Broader population
> - Can examine several standard of care therapies
> - Large number of participants ('big data'), so can see e.g. uncommon adverse events
> - Can look at long term effects (benefits)
> - Adherence to treatments might be lower (realistic) than in RCTs
> - Real-world experience (adherence, stopping treatment early and side effects) might yield a more realistic estimate of the benefits and harms of an intervention.

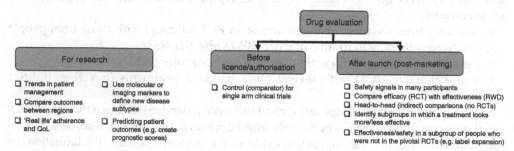

Figure 9.8 Some common proposed uses of real-world data. The uses associated with drug evaluation can be used for other intervention types. RCT, randomised controlled trial.

performance of a new car on a racing circuit, with one driver and in ideal driving conditions. While effectiveness is analogous to real life driving conditions: bumpy roads, variable weather conditions and ≥1 passenger in the car.

RWD analyses

When comparing two interventions in an RCT, participants are *randomly allocated* to one or more interventions, which by design minimises confounding and some biases. However, in a real-world setting, there may be all sorts of reasons why one person has Therapy A and another person has Therapy B, when they have the same disorder. This inherent confounding makes it difficult to compare outcomes reliably using the observed data.

Box 9.9 Main types and sources of real-world data

Types of RWD	Sources of data

Types of RWD

- Participant demographics and disease characteristics
- Interventions (and details)
- Co-morbidities
- Measures of effectiveness/ treatment response
- Adverse events (especially symptomatic)
- Patient reported outcomes (including QoL, treatment satisfaction)
- Adherence

Sources of data

- Primary:
  A (new) research project conducted by investigators, often disease-specific.
- Secondary:
  Data collected by someone else (e.g. regional/ national database or registry). Often population level, and not disease specific.
- Directly from individual hospitals/clinics
- Non-commercial/governmental/academic organisations (e.g. death/disease registries)
- Commercial organisations/payers (e.g. claims/ reimbursement/insurance databases)
- Directly from participants/patients: personal electronic devices/mobile phones, apps, wearables.

A key part of the methods for RWD analysis is to try to balance the baseline (pre-treatment) demographic and disease characteristics between the participant groups being compared. If the dataset *can be made to look like* a randomised trial, then it might be analysed and interpreted as one. The methods therefore attempt to 'model' the reasons why people are given different interventions, to produce a dataset that has balanced characteristics.

Figure 9.9 is an example of using RWD to evaluate the addition of a (then) newly approved drug (palbociclib; a first-in-class CDK4/6 inhibitor) to standard of care letrozole (an aromatase inhibitor), for treating metastatic breast cancer.[27] This is an example of comparing interventions using RWD only.

In the dataset, there are clear baseline (pre-treatment) differences for patient and disease characteristics between those who had palbociclib + letrozole versus letrozole alone, for example: age ≥75 (20 vs 38%), and performance status 2–4 which is a measure of a person's physical fitness (6 vs 13%). Outcomes should not be compared between the two groups without allowing for these differences.

In standard epidemiological case-control studies, a simple way to get balanced groups is by **matching**. For example, we would take one patient who had been given the doublet therapy (e.g. age 45 years and performance status 2), and then try to find an equivalent (or sufficiently similar) patient from the letrozole alone group. However, this is difficult to achieve with many factors.

Another approach is to perform multivariable regression analyses that produce an effect size adjusted for personal and disease characteristics, but this involves assumptions about the association between each factor and the outcome measure (e.g. they have a linear relationship), and the regression model may not function properly if there are many factors but insufficient participants.

An efficient approach is to use **propensity scores**, which essentially convert multiple factors into a single numerical measure.

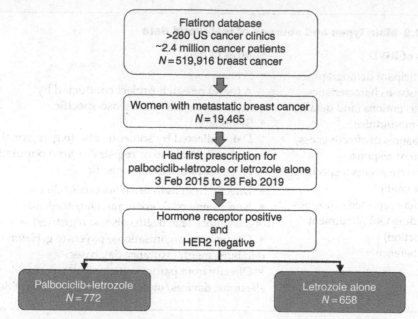

Figure 9.9 Outline of an observational study to evaluate the real-world efficacy of adding palbociclib to standard letrozole, for first-line treatment of advanced breast cancer.[27] The data source is Flatiron (a commercially owned large dataset of electronic health records prospectively collated from many cancer clinics). HER2, human epidermal growth factor receptor-negative.

The premise is that multiple factors are considered to influence the choice of treatment for an individual. Regression methods model the association between these factors and the treatment given. Figure 9.10 illustrates this. The model is derived using the dataset (e.g. 772 + 658 patients in Figure 9.9), and then applied to all trial participants to produce a propensity score for each of them: generally the chance of being given Treatment A given their characteristics, whether they actually had Treatment A or not (Box 9.10).

Once we have the propensity scores, there are several ways that they can be used, two of which are propensity score matching (PSM) and inverse probability of treatment weighting (IPTW); Figure 9.11. They are fundamentally different approaches, but they both aim to produce a dataset that has balanced characteristics, which can then be analysed and interpreted as if it came from an RCT. Applying the propensity score in this way essentially uses the person and disease factors to re-design the study to resemble an RCT *before* the analysis that produces an effect size. This is in contrast to standard multivariable analyses that maintains the study design and allows for the person and disease factors *as part of* the analysis.

PSM involves taking each person in the palbociclib + letrozole group, and then finds (matches them to) someone from the letrozole-only group who has a similar propensity score (within a sufficiently narrow range). The dataset to be analysed is often a smaller subset than the original because some participants cannot be matched.

IPTW uses the propensity score as weights that are applied to each person in the dataset (Box 9.11). This essentially creates a new dataset that often (not always) seems larger than the original dataset.

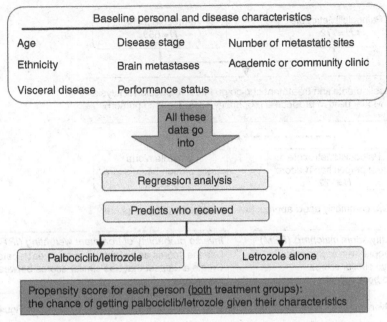

Figure 9.10 Outline of how a propensity score is obtained (based on the example in Figure 9.9).

Box 9.10 Illustration of a propensity score model and its interpretation

Hypothetically, suppose we have only age and brain metastases to consider, and the regression analysis produces the following model and coefficients:

Function of (chance of getting palbociclib + letrozole) = $-3 + 0.025 \times \underline{Age} + 0.6 \times \underline{Brain\ Mets}$ (0 if No, 1 if Yes)

Patient A is aged 52 with no brain metastases, so her raw score is $-3 + 0.025 \times \underline{52} + 0.6 \times \underline{0} = -1.7$.

This converts to a propensity score of 15%, i.e. given her age and brain metastases status the chance of being given palbociclib + letrozole is 15%.[#]

Patient B is aged 75 with brain metastases, so her raw score is $-3 + 0.025 \times \underline{75} + 0.6 \times \underline{1} = -0.52$.

This converts to a propensity score of 37%, reflecting a higher chance of getting the doublet therapy given the less favourable risk factors.

[#]Propensity score = $\exp^{raw\ score}/(1 + \exp^{raw\ score})$; exp is the exponential number 2.7183. In the example, $\exp^{-1.7}/[1 + \exp^{-1.7}] = 0.15$.

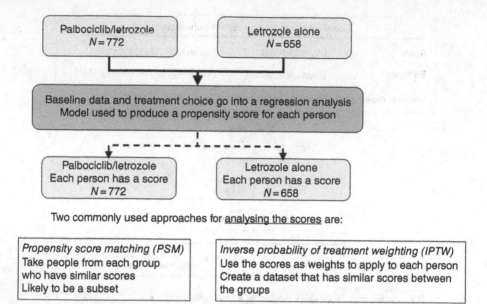

Figure 9.11 Overview of the regression modelling and how it is used (based on the example in Figure 9.9).

Box 9.11 Illustration of how weights are used in the inverse probability of treatment weighting (IPTW) approach

To illustrate how IPTW works, let us assume a person has a propensity score of 0.75 (i.e. the chance of getting palbociclib + letrozole is 3/4, so the chance of getting letrozole alone is 1/4).

This means that among four people with similar characteristics, we expect three to have doublet therapy and one has letrozole alone. This is an ideal comparison because they have the same propensity score, but there are too few who had letrozole only. So we apply the scores as weights, where each person is 'multiplied' (weighted/'cloned') by 1/ (chance of getting what they actually received).

The three who had doublet therapy are each multiplied by 1/0.75 = 1.333 [the three becomes four people, i.e. 1.333 × 3]

The one who had letrozole only is multiplied by 1/0.25 = 4 [the one person becomes four people]

The new dataset now contains four people in each group with broadly similar characteristics because they have the same propensity score.

Whichever analytical method is used, it is essential to check that the baseline characteristics have become similar. Using the IPTW method in the breast cancer example, balance was achieved for palbociclib + letrozole versus letrozole alone, for example: age ≥75 (28 vs 28%), and performance status 2–4 (10 vs 10%).[27] Figure 9.12 shows the Kaplan-Meier curves using the unadjusted comparison, and after the two methods were applied. There is good consistency in the hazard ratios, which is not always seen.

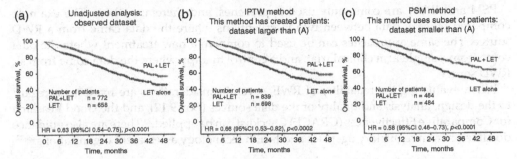

Figure 9.12 Overall survival for the example in Figure 9.9; showing the results using (a) the initial (unadjusted) analysis, (b) inverse probability of treatment weighting (IPTW) method, and (c) propensity score matching (PSM). PAL: palbociclib, LET: letrozole, HR: hazard ratio. Source: DeMichele et al.[27]/figure reproduced with permission from Springer Nature/Breast Cancer Research/ CC BY 4.0

Box 9.12 Evaluating the reliability of real-world evidence

Design	Analysis	Quality of the RWD source(s)
Are the participants representative of the target population of interest?	Have all important participant and disease confounding factors been included in the modelling?	Are the major participant and disease characteristics, and outcomes measured reliably/accurately?
Prospective or retrospective data (former is often better)?	Do the methods produce well balanced characteristics?	Are there much missing data for major variables?
Is there major bias in how participants were managed, treated, recruited to the database or selected for the specific analyses?*	Have there been sensitivity analyses (e.g. different assumptions about missing data) and do they produce consistent results?	Is there transparency in the data processing (e.g. collation of the dataset)?
Is there sufficient follow up, with sufficient events?	Do different statistical methods produce similar results?	Is there known provenance and traceability of the dataset?
Have major participant and disease characteristics (confounding factors) been measured/included?		Have appropriate data protection regulations been complied with?
Is the comparator therapy relevant to current practice?		

*Any *systematic* difference between the treatment groups being compared (e.g. patients in the new treatment arm came from tertiary/expert centres, but those in the comparator arm came from community clinics)

PSM and IPTW are commonly used approaches, and there are others. The example compared efficacy data between two interventions where the data came from a RWD source. The same approaches can be used to compare a new treatment where the data come from a single-arm clinical trial, and a control therapy where the data come from an RWD source.

When evaluating the reliability of RWE, several considerations are made with regard to the design, analysis and quality of the data sources (Box 9.12), and the Good Research for Comparative Effectiveness (GRACE) Checklist can be applied.[28] There are also guidance documents from regulatory agencies and health technology assessment organisations.[29-32]

9.4 Summary points

- Systematic reviews are based on a formal approach to obtaining, analysing and interpreting all the available studies on a particular topic
- A meta-analysis combines all relevant studies to give a single estimate of the effect size, which usually (not always) has greater precision than any individual trial
- The conclusions from a review are usually stronger than those from any single study.
- Meta-analyses can be used for direct and indirect treatment comparisons.
- Real-world data and real-world evidence can provide good supporting evidence alongside randomised trials, and also data in the absence of randomised studies for uncommon/rare disorders, although care is required for their interpretation and how confounding and bias have been handled.

References

1. Davey Smith G, Egger M, Phillips AN. Meta-analysis: beyond the grand mean? *BMJ* 1997; **315**:1610–1614.
2. Egger M, Davey Smith G. Meta-analysis: potentials and promise. *BMJ* 1997; **315**:1371–1374.
3. Egger M, Davey Smith G. Meta-analysis: bias in location and selection of studies. *BMJ* 1998; **316**:61–66.
4. Egger M, Davey Smith G, Phillips AN. Meta-analysis: principles and procedures. *BMJ* 1997; **315**:1533–1537.
5. Egger M, Davey Smith G, Schneider M, Minder CE. Bias in meta-analysis detected by a simple graphical test. *BMJ* 1997; **315**: 629–634.
6. Egger M, Schneider M, Davey Smith G. Meta-analysis: spurious precision? Meta-analysis of observational studies. *BMJ* 1998; **316**:140–144.
7. Glasziou P, Irwig L, Bain C, Colditz G. *Systematic Reviews in Health Care: A Practical Guide*. Cambridge University Press, 2008.
8. Egger M, Davey Smith G, Altman D. (Eds). *Systematic Reviews in Health Care: Meta-analysis in Context*, 2nd edn, BMJ Books, 2001.
9. Khan KS, Kunz R, Kleijnen J, Antes G. *Systematic Reviews to Support Evidence-based Medicine: How to Review and Apply Findings of Healthcare Research*. Royal Society of Medicine Press Ltd, 2003.
10. Pammi M, Suresh G. Enteral lactoferrin supplementation for prevention of sepsis and necrotizing enterocolitis in preterm infants. *Cochrane Database Syst Rev.* 2017; 6 (CD007137)
11. ELFIN trial investigators group. Enteral lactoferrin supplementation for very preterm infants: a randomised placebo-controlled trial Lancet 2019;393(10170):423–433
12. https://handbook-5-1.cochrane.org/part_2_general_methods_for_cochrane_reviews.htm.

13. Tang JL, Law M, Wald N. How effective is nicotine replacement therapy in helping people to stop smoking? *BMJ* 1994; **308**:21–26.

14. RevMan. https://revman.cochrane.org/info.

15. Higgins JPT, Thompson SG, Deeks JJ, Altman DG. Measuring inconsistency in meta-analyses. *BMJ* 2003; **327**:557–560.

16. DerSimonian R, Laird N. Meta-analysis in clinical trials. *Control Clin Trials* 1986; **7**:177–188.

17. Spiro SG, James LE, Rudd RM *et al.*; London Lung Cancer Group. Early compared with late radiotherapy in combined modality treatment for limited disease small-cell lung cancer: a London Lung Cancer Group multicenter randomized clinical trial and meta-analysis. *J Clin Oncol* 2006; 24(24):3823–3830.

18. Sterne JAC, Egger M, Davey Smith G. Systematic reviews in health care: investigating and dealing with publication and other biases in meta-analysis. *BMJ* 2001; **323**:101–105.

19. Page MJ, McKenzie JE, Bossuyt PM *et al*. The PRISMA 2020 statement: an updated guideline for reporting systematic reviews. *BMJ* 2021; 372:n71. doi: https://doi.org/10.1136/bmj.n71.

20. Hutton B, Salanti G, Caldwell DM *et al*. The PRISMA extension statement for reporting of systematic reviews incorporating network meta-analyses of health care interventions: checklist and explanations. *Ann Intern Med* 2015; **162**(11):777–784.

21. Zhao Y, Liu J, Cai X *et al*. Efficacy and safety of first line treatments for patients with advanced epidermal growth factor receptor mutated, non-small cell lung cancer: systematic review and network meta-analysis. *BMJ* 2019; 367:l5460.

22. Collins R, MacMahon S. Reliable assessment of the effects of treatment on mortality and major morbidity, I: clinical trials. *Lancet* 2001; 357:373–380.

23. Sherman RE, Anderson SA, Dal Pan GJ *et al*. Real-world evidence – what is it and what can it tell us? *N Engl J Med* 2016; **375**(23):2293–2297.

24. Cave A, Kurz X, Arlett P. Real-world data for regulatory decision making: challenges and possible solutions for Europe. *Clin Pharmacol Ther* 2019; **106**(1):36–39.

25. Concato J, Corrigan-Curay J. Real-world evidence – where are we now? *N Engl J Med* 2022; **386**(18):1680–1682.

26. Corrigan-Curay J, Sacks L, Woodcock J. Real-world evidence and real-world data for evaluating drug safety and effectiveness. *JAMA* 2018; **320**(9):867–868.

27. DeMichele A, Cristofanilli M, Brufsky A *et al*. Comparative effectiveness of first-line palbociclib plus letrozole versus letrozole alone for HR+/HER2- metastatic breast cancer in US real-world clinical practice. *Breast Cancer Res* 2021; **23**(1):37. doi: https://doi.org/10.1186/s13058-021-01409-8.

28. Dreyer NA, Velentgas P, Westrich K, Dubois R. The GRACE checklist for rating the quality of observational studies of comparative effectiveness: a tale of hope and caution J Manag Care Spec Pharm. 2014;20(3):301–8

29. European Medicines Agency Real-world evidence framework to support EU regulatory decision-making. Report on the experience gained with regulator-led studies from September 2021 to February 2023. https://www.ema.europa.eu/system/files/documents/report/real-world-evidence-framework-support-eu-regulatory-decision-making-report-experience-gained_en.pdf

30. US Food and Drug Administration. Considerations for the design and conduct of externally controlled trials for drug and biological products. 2023. https://www.fda.gov/regulatory-information/search-fda-guidance-documents/considerations-design-and-conduct-externally-controlled-trials-drug-and-biological-products

31. National Institute for Health and Care Excellence. NICE real-world evidence framework. 2022. https://www.nice.org.uk/corporate/ecd9/chapter/overview

32. Wang SV, Pottegård A, Crown W, et al. Harmonized protocol template to enhance reproducibility of hypothesis evaluating real-world evidence studies on treatment effects: a good practices report of a joint ISPE/ISPOR task force. Pharmacoepidemiol Drug Saf. 2023;32(1):44–55

CHAPTER 10

Conducting and reporting trials

Setting up and conducting clinical trials require a concerted collaboration between people with different but complementary roles across several organisations. The multiple procedures and documents required can appear daunting, even for what should be relatively simple studies. There are national regulations that apply to all types of interventions and additional ones specific to investigational medicinal products (drugs) and some medical devices, and guidelines on best practices. Current regulatory requirements should always be checked as they are periodically updated. Institutions (sponsors) often have their own internal processes and procedures. This chapter outlines the clinical trial process in general (Figure 10.1). At the end is a section on why trials 'fail'.

It is a useful exercise to consider the conduct of a clinical trial from the view point of the participants (e.g. appeal of the trial interventions and how they are given/administered, how easy the study assessments are and their frequency, and the ability to get to healthcare facilities for either the interventions or assessments). Any of these can influence trial uptake, adherence and withdrawing from the trial. Working closely with patient/public representatives can help identify potential issues and mitigate them before the trial is launched.

10.1 Working group and key roles

A small multidisciplinary **working group** of key people (say, three to five) should initially develop the project. They agree on the trial objectives, design and outcome measures, and share responsibility for writing the trial protocol and, perhaps, the grant application. The group should include health professionals, a statistician, patient/public representative(s), and other speciality members, e.g., trial co-ordinator, pathologist or health economist.

Once the trial has been funded, the group can expand to form the **Trial Management Group**, or **Trial Steering Group/Committee** to oversee the trial. Additional expertise might include data management, regulations, pharmacovigilance and safety monitoring, IT (database and randomisation systems), and investigators from some of the larger recruiting centres. There are a few key specific roles (Box 10.1).

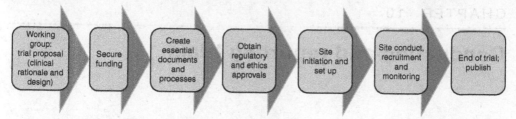

Figure 10.1 High-level overview of a typical clinical trial process.

Box 10.1 Key roles involved in a clinical trial

Sponsor: an organisation that has ultimate (and legal) responsibility for the trial, to ensure that it is conducted in accordance with relevant regulations and guidelines. A sponsor can be the manufacturer of a drug (pharmaceutical company) or medical device, a university, a hospital or a healthcare facility.

Chief, principal or lead investigator: a named health professional with oversight of the trial. They often conceived the trial proposal, and are key opinion leaders in the disease area or senior employees of the sponsor. They are usually the first point of contact for regulatory and ethics committee issues, and other major problems that arise; and are the signatory for important documents.

Principal or site investigator: a named health professional who is responsible for the trial at a particular centre (site) that recruits or manages trial participants.

10.2 Estimate and secure funding

Staff funding and resources necessary to set up and conduct a trial should not be under-estimated. The number and type of central staff required will depend on the complexity of the trial but often include a co-ordinator, data manager, statistician, and database programmer. This is in addition to running expenses such as office, printing, and travel costs for investigator meetings and visiting sites. For medicinal products/drugs and some medical devices, costs of submissions to regulatory agencies for a clinical trial approval and any future amendments also need to be included.

Large trials often require full-time dedicated staff, but small trials, where there are few participants recruited per month from a few centres may only require part of a person's time. Costs incurred by a recruiting site could include:

- A fee for each participant recruited to cover identifying potential participants, perform eligibility assessments, take consent, administer the trial interventions that are not standard of care, plan trial-specific visits, data management (data entry and checking), and adverse event reporting.
- Those for clinical assessments, blood or tissue samples, pathological reviews or laboratory analyses that are in addition to standard practice

Pharmaceutical and medical device companies fund and sponsor many trials (e.g. studies for regulatory marketing authorisation/licence and market access), and they also fund academic-sponsored studies (investigator-initiated trials). Non-commercial organisations usually require external funding that comes from governmental or international funding agencies, charities and private benefactors. Grant applications are competitive and relatively few succeed, hence they need to be written clearly and represent value for money.[1] They are more likely to be successful if the trial has the potential to change practice, provides valuable insight into how a disorder is treated, or represents a novel intervention.

10.3 Patient and Public Involvement and Engagement (PPIE)

PPIE is now an expected and essential component of clinical trial design, delivery and interpretation.[2,3] One or more representatives could:
- Help with the trial design (e.g. whether the new treatment looks appealing to them, whether the control therapy is appropriate, and whether the trial-specific clinic visits/assessments are too many or arduous).
- Help design and write the participant-facing materials, videos, and webpage, in order to make them more readable and therefore increase trial accrual and retention.
- Be a key member of the Trial Management/Steering Group, and help to identify and propose solutions for problems with recruitment and conduct.
- Help interpret the results and conclusions, which can form materials to be sent to the participants and to disease-specific organisations (patient charities and support groups).
- Be members of the independent oversight committees (e.g. DSMB/IDMC, see page 187).

Patients and lay members often see a clinical trial from a different but complementary perspective than the health professional investigators.

Many grant funding organisations expect to see evidence of PPIE input from the start, and not just from a single person but rather several representatives. Without significant input, grant applications may be less likely to be successful. Collaborating with a disease-specific charity or patient support group can provide excellent input. One situation where this is especially useful is to get a range of acceptable non-inferiority margins for a non-inferiority trial.

10.4 Essential trial documents

Figure 10.2 shows several documents and key processes required for a typical clinical trial, and these are each covered in the numbered sections in this chapter. The documents are outlined in the following sections.

Trial protocol[4]

The protocol (Box 10.2) provides the justification for the trial; the design; a set of instructions for sites and the co-ordinating centre describing how participants are to be recruited and followed up, and the trial interventions administered; and the systems in place for monitoring adverse events (Box 10.2). It ensures the trial is conducted to a similar standard across all sites. The protocol is signed off by the sponsor and chief investigator. Although the protocol should contain all the necessary information to allow sites to conduct the study with minimal queries, an overly long document can be difficult to implement and comply with, and may therefore deter sites from taking part.

Eligibility criteria should be worded clearly (to avoid sites constantly querying their definition with the sponsor) and carefully, in order to avoid numerous eligibility waivers and deviations (see page 185) that may attract criticism. Essential criteria could have

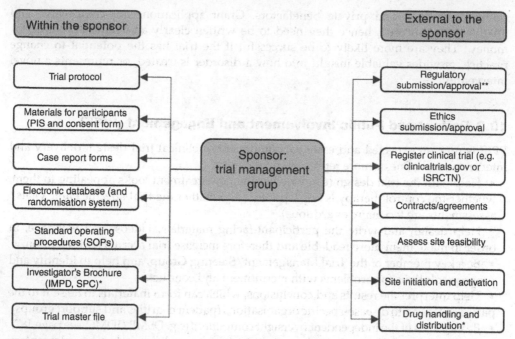

Figure 10.2 Overview of essential documents and processes used for setting up a typical trial. The protocol, PIS, consent form, and Investigators Brochure/IMPD/SPC are needed for the regulatory and ethics approvals. *Required for trials of investigational drugs and some medical devices. **Investigational New Drug application (US, Canada, Japan), Clinical Trial Application (Europe, UK). IMPD, Investigational Medicinal Product Dossier; SPC, Summary of Product Characteristics; PIS, Participant Information Sheet; ISRCTN, International Standard Randomized Controlled Trial Number.

strict wording ('must'), while others are described to allow some flexibility when deciding who to recruit ('could').

A schedule of assessments (Table 10.1) that is clear and easy for site staff to follow, also makes it easier to estimate the trial cost including costs to be paid to sites. The timing of QoL assessments depends on the natural course of the disorder and when detectable changes in QoL are expected to occur (e.g. every 3 months for a trial of an advanced disorder where most patients die within 1–2 years, or every 12 months in a disease prevention trial among healthy people).

Clinical trial regulations apply to any medicinal product (and some medical devices) specified in the protocol, even if it is not actually being evaluated (e.g. it could be a background standard of care given to all participants). However, if the protocol does not mandate such drugs and their administration, and just indicates that clinics have to deliver the standard of care therapy,# it could mean that the study is not covered by the regulations. This will make the trial easier to run.

Participant/Patient Information Sheet (PIS) and Consent Form

A PIS provides the necessary information to eligible participants so that they can make an informed choice whether to enrol in the trial or not. The PIS covers items in Box 10.3, ideally using simple language, and it sometimes needs to be available in multiple languages (e.g. international trials). The front cover of a full PIS could contain a very short

---

There could just be a list of standard therapies that are commonly used.

Box 10.2 General sections in a typical trial protocol

Section heading	Description
Chief investigator and Sponsor	• Name and address of one individual who is the overall lead, and the representative of the institution acting as the sponsor • Both need to sign and date each version
Trial management	• Names, affiliations and roles
Background	• A fairly concise summary of the disease burden (e.g. prevalence or incidence) and effect of current treatments, with reference to appropriate studies or systematic reviews
Justification for the trial	• A summary of why a trial is needed now, and how it may be expected to change practice, used to justify further studies, or provide additional knowledge • Current evidence and biological plausibility for the new intervention
Trial design	• Type of trial— phase I, II or III; randomised or single-arm; single- or double-blind; biomarker-directed study
Objectives	• One or two primary objectives, and several secondary ones to provide additional information
Outcome measures	• Each endpoint should be quantitative and correspond to an objective
Target population	• A clearly defined list of the inclusion and exclusion criteria
Interventions	• A clear description of what the trial interventions are and how they will be administered, and any modifications following adverse events • Other treatments to be given at the same time should be indicated • If free drugs or medical devices are supplied, a summary of how they will be supplied and (if appropriate) unused medicines destroyed
Consent	• Summarise the procedures for obtaining informed consent
Recruitment and Follow-up	• Specify the length of the accrual and follow-up periods (added together they represent the total trial length)
Assessments of participants	• Details of how participants will be assessed: duration and frequency, and what happens to them at each visit
Case report forms	• When they are administered and who completes them: participant or researcher
Safety monitoring	• A list of any known expected adverse reactions associated with the trial treatments • Describe the procedures for identifying, monitoring and reporting adverse events
Sample size	• There should be enough information for the sample size to be reproduced independently, with reference to the expected treatment effects from published or unpublished work, or a target effect that is the least clinically important
Statistical analyses	• Outline of the statistical methods (primary and secondary outcomes); type of analysis (e.g. intention-to-treat or per-protocol); interim and subgroup analyses; handling censoring and missing data
Insurance and indemnity	• What cover is in place if a person is harmed through participating in the trial
Ownership	• A statement about ownership of the trial data
Biospecimens	• A section (or appendix) outlining what biospecimens are to be collected: when, how the site has to process, store and ship them, and where they need to be sent

Table 10.1 Example of a table that summarises the schedule (timing) of assessments of participants.

	Baseline	Intervention period (therapy is given for 12 months)			Follow-up	
		3 months	6	12	18	24
Assessments						
Medical history	X					
Clinical examination	X	X	X	X	X	X
Blood sample	X			X		X
Imaging scan	X			X		
Quality of life questionnaire	X		X	X		X

Box 10.3 Recommended sections in a Participant Information Sheet (PIS)

• Background and justification for the trial.
• How participants would be randomised (if relevant), and the probability of being in each trial arm.
• A description of the trial interventions, especially identifying those that are experimental.
• What the participant has to do as part of the trial (e.g. extra clinic visits, scans or assessments), and the expected duration of their participation.
• Which biospecimens are collected, and their purpose.
• What are the possible side-effects of the interventions.
• The possible benefits and disadvantages of taking part.
• A statement about securing confidentiality of participants' data and who will have access to the data, including data sharing with collaborators.
• A statement that participation is voluntary and refusal to participate will involve no penalty or loss of care; and that the participant may withdraw at any time.
• Who is funding the research.
• Who to contact if there are any queries, including a 24-hour telephone number in an emergency.
• A statement about liability and compensation if something goes wrong.

---

and simple outline of why the study is being done, the trial interventions, and what participants need to do during the trial.

Modern approaches for creating a PIS include using cartoons and short online videos perhaps with animations to complement the fuller PIS. This can make the trial materials more understandable by a wider group (e.g. ethnic minorities, the elderly, those with mental or physical disabilities, and those from socially disadvantaged backgrounds or lower educational levels). Many PIS are overly long with 'high level' (e.g. graduate level) or technical language, so potential participants either do not understand the study or they do not find it appealing enough to enrol.

The PIS can be on paper or accessible electronically via personal devices (e.g. mobile phones, notepads and laptops) and involve electronic signatures.

> **Box 10.4 Examples of text used in a consent form**
>
> • I confirm that I have read and understood the information sheet Version 1.0 dated 10 January 2023.
> • I understand that my participation is voluntary and that I am free to withdraw at any time, without giving any reason and without my medical care or legal rights being affected.
> • I understand that my medical notes may be looked at by responsible individuals or by regulatory authorities where it is relevant to my taking part in research.
> • I give permission for extra blood/urine/tissue samples to be taken during the trial. I understand that giving these samples is voluntary.
> • I agree that the samples I have given, and the information gathered about me, can be stored for use in future research and with other collaborators, even if I withdraw from the trial procedures.
> • I agree for my family physician to be told of my participation in this study.
> • I agree to participate in the trial.
> • Signature of the participant or legal guardian.

Creative PIS pamphlets and online videos can contain testimonials from and feature people with the disorder of interest (e.g. trial participants) talking about their positive experiences. Sponsors could place the materials on their website, where they can be easily accessed, and include regular trial updates.

Informed consent is a legal requirement, and participants should be allowed sufficient time to consider the trial. There is usually no rule over what is considered a minimum time; consent can be given on the same day or a few days after the PIS. A consent form (Box 10.4) is required to show that the person has received and understood the trial materials and has decided to take part. In some circumstances where direct consent is not possible (e.g. paediatric/childhood disorders, emergency hospital admissions, or the person is unconscious or temporarily incapacitated) an attending clinician and (where possible) a legal representative of the participant (parent, close relative or guardian) can give consent. If an adult becomes aware later on, they may be asked to re-consent.

In geographically diverse trials, including in developing countries where educational levels in rural areas may be low, the consent process could be recorded on video (e.g. mobile phone or tablet). Many trials have used paper consent forms, but this can involve an additional visit to the clinic after reading the PIS. Electronic consent forms (E-consent) are increasingly used, via personal devices, mobile phone apps or accessing a weblink, and this can be done from home.

Paper versions of the PIS and consent form should still be available for those who request them.

Case report forms (CRFs)

Data can come from various sources (see Box 1.5 page 11). CRFs contain specific items of information about participants, required to monitor the trial and for all analyses.

Main types of CRFs include baseline characteristics (demographics and disease features), treatment details, efficacy outcomes, QoL and safety. Baseline information on ethnicity/race, and markers of socioeconomic background (e.g. educational level, profession, income, home address) can be collected to see whether enrolled participants are representative of a wider group.

CRFs should be easy to understand, and simple and relatively quick to complete. They should always be tested on a few people first before launching them. Having many variables, particularly in phase III trials, may result in complex or multiple forms, and site staff may not complete key variables. *Many trials collect too much data that are never analysed*.

Some trials use paper CRFs that are completed for each participant by research staff and posted to the central coordinating centre, where they are manually entered into an electronic database. **Electronic data capture systems (eCRFs)** are efficient and allow personnel at study sites to enter data directly into the central database.

The use of personal electronic devices and wearables allow real-time collection of data (e.g. efficacy, side effects, adherence, QoL, and satisfaction with the interventions) directly from participants, so that they spend less time in clinics providing this information. Remote clinical assessments (telephone or video-conferencing) can also replace some in-person clinic visits.

Electronic database (randomisation system)

Trial data are entered into an electronic database (either bespoke or commercial). This ensures that data entry is structured making it easier to check and correct data, and analyse. For trials of investigational medicines, the database should be validated, and have an **audit trail** of activity, where changes to the data are recorded. Automated validation checks can minimise data entry error, or identify errors on the CRFs that need correcting (e.g. date of death comes before the date of starting trial treatment). Range checks identify extreme blood and physiological measurements to be checked. The database may help identify overdue CRFs, or missing key variables.

Database systems must be secure, with access limited to relevant staff, and backed up regularly. For double-blind trials, treatment allocation should only be visible in the database as a drug pack code so that trial staff with regular access cannot see which intervention has been allocated to each participant.

For randomised trials, a reliable system is needed that randomly allocates the trial interventions, and incorporates participants' details that are used as stratification factors (see Box 1.4, page 10). Such systems can be created or are already within commercial database software.

Standard operating procedures (SOPs)

These ensure that trials are conducted to a consistent standard within the coordinating centre (sponsor) and across study sites. They show staff how to perform certain functions and allow new staff to familiarise themselves with these practices. SOPs also show an external auditor or regulatory inspector that clear and robust systems are in place. Examples of SOPs are:

- How to develop the protocol, and templates for the PIS and consent form
- Making and reporting protocol amendments
- How to prepare and submit for regulatory and ethics approvals
- Assessing the feasibility of sites and how to set them up
- Development and maintenance of the database and randomisation systems
- Data management: how to check and chase up key data fields
- Handling adverse events, protocol violations and serious breaches
- Site visits during the trial

- Monitoring and risk assessment plans for participants and sites
- Statistical considerations (sample size, statistical analysis plan)
- Closing the trial (chasing missing data, ensuring that all the trial documentation is stored).

Investigator's Brochure (IB)

This provides detailed information about any trial investigational medicinal product whether it already has a licence/marketing authorisation or not, including its chemical, toxicological, pharmacological and safety properties, and dose and method of delivery, with evidence from laboratory and animal studies. It allows trial investigators to assess the possible risks and benefits of the drug. There should be one IB for each drug being evaluated, and it is not usually specific to a trial.

For drugs already licensed for human use, and to be used within the terms of its marketing authorisation, a regulatory body may require a **Summary of Product Characteristics** (SPC) instead of a detailed IB. The **Investigational Medicinal Product Dossier (IMPD;** EU IMP trials) provides information about the quality, safety and use of all IMPs in the trial, including placebo or any other comparator. It allows the regulatory body to examine the possible toxicity profile of the product(s). Some information will overlap with that in the IB, and so can simply be cross-referenced. Again, the SPC may suffice for drugs already licensed for human use.

The IB, SPC and IMPD are developed and updated by the drug manufacturer, who should also provide an example of the drug label for its packaging.

Trial Master File (TMF)

This consists of all the key documents either kept in a single physical location (paper files) or electronically (eTMF). At the sponsor's office, it includes the Investigator's Brochure (IB) or equivalent (for drug trials), all protocol versions, all versions of the PIS and consent forms, indemnification and insurance documents, all necessary approval documents that have been received, signed contracts and agreements, and curriculum vitae for the key investigators. At study sites, the TMF includes a staff delegation log (listing everyone involved in conducting the trial), key communications with the sponsor, and serious adverse event reports. TMFs are updated during the trial.

10.5 Ethics and regulatory approvals

All trials require independent ethics approval, and in addition studies of medicinal products and some medical devices require regulatory approval; Figure 10.2. These approvals are required in each country (or the EU) in which the trial would be conducted, and the processes and requirements should be checked as they are revised periodically.

Ethics approval

This involves an Institutional Review Board (IRB) or Research Ethics Committee (REC) from an independent formally recognised organisation that could be within a hospital or university, or a regional or national body. The IRB/REC examines the trial protocol, and any materials intended for participants (e.g. PIS, consent form, videos and self-completed questionnaires). These are contained in an application form submitted by the trial sponsor. The IRB/REC consists of a group of scientific experts and lay members who consider the justification for the trial and its design; acceptability to participants, including the potential harms and benefits, and any major ethical issues; and procedures for compensating participants in case of negligence.

Applications are stronger if the trial has already been independently peer reviewed (e.g. through a grant application), and if patient or public representatives have been closely involved in the study design and creation of the participant-facing materials.

The IRB/REC may request changes to the trial design, conduct or documentation. The process for obtaining ethical approval varies between countries and according to whether the trial is single or multi-centre. For multi-centre studies, national approval might be possible (e.g. the UK), allowing the trial to be conducted anywhere in that location. In the US, there may be one IRB at each recruiting site, or one that covers several sites.

There is usually a time limit for the review. In several places, the target is typically 60 days to approve or decline the application, with extra time if changes are requested.

Regulatory approval

In most countries, national regulations focus on trials of an investigational medicinal product. Generally, a substance, or combination of substances, is an IMP/IND if the trial aims to determine whether it affects disease treatment, detection or diagnosis, or prevents disease or early death. In some countries, it may also include substances used to restore, correct or modify physiological functions (e.g. in the EU). Regulatory approvals may also be required for some medical devices and radioactive exposures.

Each country has its own agency to issue regulatory approval to allow trials to be conducted (see Table 8.1, page 128). In the EU, the EU-CTR (EU Clinical Trial Regulation 536/2014) allows a centralised and single National Competent Authority (NCA) and Ethics Committee (EC) application to be submitted, followed by a single decision across all EU member states. This is done through the Clinical Trial Information System (CTIS) portal and database, and should significantly streamline clinical trial approvals across the EU. In the US, the application is done through the FDA portal.

To gain regulatory approval, several documents and information must be submitted electronically (Box 10.5): called a **Clinical Trial Application** (CTA, in the EU), or **Investigational New Drug application** (in the US). This is reviewed by a panel of experts who will approve the trial if it appears to be sufficiently safe for participants, and the benefit–harm balance is likely to be favourable.

Box 10.5 Typical information needed for submission for regulatory approval to conduct a drug trial

- Investigator's Brochure (IB); Summary of Product Characteristics (SPC) Investigational Medicinal Product Dossier (IMPD), each where relevant
- Preclinical studies, and dose-finding studies, toxicology and pharmacology information in humans
- Details of drug manufacturing, quality control and distribution (e.g. Qualified Person documentation in the EU)
- Trial protocol, Participant Information Sheet and consent form
- Information about the investigators, recruiting sites and laboratories
- Specification of measures to deal with vulnerable participants, when required

---

It is sometimes useful to meet with the regulators to reach agreement on the trial design, particularly for phase III trials to be used for a marketing authorisation application. In the US, sponsors could arrange a formal meeting with the FDA. In the EU, sponsors may seek scientific advice from the Committee for Medicinal Products for Human Use (CHMP).

Regulatory authorities typically aim to assess applications in about 30 days, but this is extended if further information is requested. For some trials, e.g. gene therapy, genetically modified organisms, or xenogenic cell therapy (live cells or tissue from animal sources to be given to humans), the approval process is longer.

10.6 Trial set up

Many academic research departments and clinical trials units have the primary purpose to design, set up and analyse clinical trials, where the host institution (university or hospital is the sponsor). Pharmaceutical companies often have an internal team. Organisations may have permanent staff in place, including clinicians, statisticians, trial coordinators, data managers, monitors and IT/database personnel. Where there is limited direct access to such resources, it is advisable to seek advice or collaborate with people who have trials experience. Many pharmaceutical companies employ a commercial contract research organisation (CRO) to set up and conduct the trial on their behalf, but the company is still the sponsor. Staff working directly on the trial, within the sponsor or recruiting sites, are expected to have certified training in Good Clinical Practice (GCP); see Section 10.11.

Register the trial

All trials need to be listed on a recognised database before recruitment starts, and this is a legal requirement in several countries. Common trial registers are:
- International Standard Randomised Controlled Trial Number (ISRCTN) (http://www.controlled-trials.com/)
- www.ClinicalTrials.gov.

These databases contain information about the main objectives, design, outcome measures, duration and funding. Many medical journals require the registration number when considering an article.

Contracts and agreements

What was once straightforward has become complicated, laborious and one of the main reasons why trials are delayed when being set up. There is a suite of agreements and legally binding contracts that are either required or requested. It is not unusual for the contracting parties to each have formal legal reviews of the documents through an external law firm (which often takes time and has an added cost). Box 10.6 outlines types of agreements (most are between the Sponsor and an external organisation).

Indemnity, liability and insurance are key items, i.e. who takes responsibility when something major goes wrong, and who has to pay compensation if this is arises (e.g. if participants have been harmed due to negligence by site staff or a major error in the trial protocol; or there has been a data breach involving personal data). Many contracts limit the amount of money that can be claimed by each party.

Investigator-initiated trials involve collaborations between academic institutions (the sponsor) and pharmaceutical companies (who provide free trial drugs and often

Box 10.6 Types of contracts and agreements used in clinical trials between the Sponsor and another party (the labels and definitions are not standard); not all are required for all studies

Type of document	Other party	Contents (most will list the roles/ responsibilities of the Sponsor)
Clinical trial site agreement*	Each recruiting site	Responsibilities of the local investigator and sites; including the responsibilities of pharmacies at sites. For international sites, it can take many months to finalise because of issues over insurance, indemnity and which country's law takes precedence.
Trial drug supply agreement	Drug/device manufacturer (often a pharmaceutical company)	Responsibilities over packaging and distribution; and that the manufacturer operates to the principles of Good Manufacturing Practice. When a commercial company is funding an academic-sponsored trial, the agreement may also contain the grant and payment details.
Quality (technical) agreement	Drug/device manufacturer	Responsibilities over manufacturing, and quality control systems are in place.
Technical/ service/third party agreement	External laboratory or organisation providing a paid-for service	Responsibilities over how biospecimens are handled, processed, stored and analysed; or outline of the service being provided. Usually no issues over data ownership and IP.
Laboratory agreement**	External laboratory is a research collaborator	Responsibilities over how biospecimens are handled, processed, stored and analysed; also include clauses about ownership of results and IP.
Material transfer agreement (MTA)	Any external party (often a formal collaborator)	Specifies what biospecimens are being sent, how they are shipped and stored, and specific analyses allowed; includes clauses about ownership of results and IP.
Data sharing agreement (DSA)		Specifies what clinical data (including scan images) are being sent; whether anonymised or not, and if not clauses over data protection are needed.

*Mandatory for EU/UK IMP trials.
**Usually for academic-sponsored trials.
IP, intellectual property.

funding). The trial concept often originated from the academic investigators. In addition to indemnity and liability, the following clauses are important:

- Data ownership
- Access by the company to the raw trial data at the end, and conditions of its use
- Inventions, intellectual property and potential for commercialisation by either party
- Being able to publish without delay or undue influence by the company.

Assess site feasibility

Potential recruiting sites may be assessed by the central trial team, to examine the local staff, systems and procedures in place for:

- Recruitment
- Storage and supply of trial drugs, medical devices or other therapy
- Administering the trial interventions and undertaking assessments
- Data collection and completion of case report forms
- Reporting adverse events.

The purpose is to identify problems that may arise, to judge whether the site is able to conduct the trial according to Good Clinical Practice (i.e. a form of **risk assessment)**, and to check that sufficient participants can be recruited. Sites also need to be content that they have enough local resources and that they will receive sufficient financial payments to conduct the trial.

Site initiation and activation

Site initiation aims to familiarise local site staff with the proposed trial and the protocol, and to establish a link with the trial co-ordination centre. The coordinator may attend the site in person, or initiation may be performed by a videoconference, particularly for relatively simple trials. Site staff involved in the study, and their delegated functions would be recorded on a **trial delegation log**.

Handling and distribution of trial drugs

The sponsor has ultimate responsibility for how investigational drugs, placebo and any other comparator drugs are sourced, manufactured, transported, stored and processed during the trial. Several procedures need to be established (Box 10.7). Some of these requirements are fulfilled by a pharmaceutical company that is supplying the trial drugs. When hospitals use their own stocks to supply licensed drugs as trial treatments, their pharmacies must have systems to record when trial drugs are dispensed to participants, including identifiers such as batch numbers. Generally, trial drugs that are used as per their licence require less oversight and monitoring.

Requirements for handling investigational drugs differ between countries. In the US, the sponsor often deals with drug quality assurance, handling and distribution, or one of more of these functions may be delegated. In the EU, IMP manufacturers or importers must hold a **manufacturing authorisation**, granted through the regulatory authority. Only the authorised holder can be involved in production, import, assembly, blinding, packaging, labelling, quality control, batch release and shipping. At least one named **Qualified Person (QP)** should be responsible for these activities. They must sign a release certificate (**QP release**) for each batch and for the final product sent to sites or trial participants. For IMPs imported into the EU, the QP must sign a QP release certificate,

---

Box 10.7 Typical quality assurance requirements of investigational drugs in clinical trials

The Sponsor should have documentation to ensure that:
• The drugs are manufactured in accordance with guidelines on Good Manufacturing Practice
• The drugs are stored according to the manufacturer's specification
• The drugs are packaged and shipped in such a way as to prevent contamination and deterioration
• Individual packages are correctly labelled (including contact details of a trial representative, expiry date, an identifier, batch number and instructions to the trial participant on storage and administration, 'keep out of reach of children' for drugs to be taken at home and 'for clinical trial use only')
• The correct pack code is given to drugs in blind trials, and that the code for a particular pack can be unbroken in an emergency in some trials
• Drugs are delivered to sites or participants in a timely fashion, and there is a clear system for ordering further supplies
• Each recruiting site keeps records on drug shipment (including dates and batch numbers) and receipt, and return and destruction of unused drugs
• Records are kept on biochemical analyses of sample batches
• Enough drugs will be available for the whole trial and target number of participants
• Drugs batches can be recalled when necessary

---

indicating that each batch meets the appropriate standards for Good Manufacturing Practice. A system may be needed to recall batches if there is a problem, particularly if drugs do not have a marketing license.

A manufacturing authorisation, QP and QP release are always needed for unlicensed drugs in the EU. QP release is not required for trial drugs that are already licensed and available from the hospital pharmacy, but it is usually required if the sponsor intends to make changes to the packaging or labelling (for example, blinding).

Handling and shipping of biospecimens or imaging scans

If translational research is part of the protocol, clear systems and processes need to be outlined for sites explaining how to process, label and ship biospecimens to a central laboratory, or how to send scan images electronically (none of which should normally contain personal identifiers such as names and dates of birth). There also need to be similarly clear processes for the central laboratory on how to receive and store biospecimens. The investigators may also specify which validated tests, assays or reagents must be used.

10.7 Conducting the trial

Once all the necessary approvals and contracts are in place sites can start to identify potential participants. Figure 10.3 shows the main trial activities.

An eligibility checklist with each of the inclusion and exclusion criteria for a participant can be 'checked off' to make clear that the person is eligible. When discussing the trial with an eligible participant, the health professional should try to maintain a position of

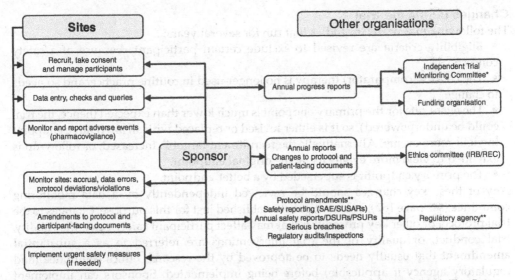

Figure 10.3 Key typical activities during a trial. ** Only required for drug or medical device trials. *E.g. Data and Safety Monitoring Board (DSMB) or Independent Data Monitoring Committee (IDMC). IRB, Institutional Review Board; REC, Research Ethics Committee; SAE, serious adverse event; SUSARs, suspected unexpected serious adverse reaction; DSUR, Development Safety Update Report; PSUR, Periodic Safety Update Report (DSURs and PSURs evaluate safety information collected during a specific reporting period, for a particular trial drug).

equipoise, i.e. there is genuine uncertainty over the effect of the new intervention. Sometimes, this is difficult to do. For example, in surgical trials, patients sometimes expect the surgeon to recommend the best treatment. Here, it might be better for another health professional to discuss the study.

In trials of medicinal products and some medical devices, participants who have consented could be given a card to carry showing their unique trial number, a brief description of the trial and 24-hour contact details of trial staff or site representatives. This is common in blind trials.

Increasing diversity within trials

Many clinical trials over the years have had a general preponderance of participants who were Caucasians (white), male, educated, younger, and those with no/few comorbidities. Trials have therefore been criticised for not being sufficiently representative of the group of people who would actually receive the intervention in practice, and that treatment efficacy might be over-estimated occasionally. To address this issue, investigators could implement ways to encourage other groups of participants to enrol in trials. The gender balance is much better generally, but there is still insufficient representation of other demographic groups (older, ethnic minorities, people from a lower socioeconomic background/socially disadvantaged, and those with disabilities). Increasing uptake in these groups can be achieved by ensuring the language in the PIS is very simple, using cartoons and short videos, and engaging with patient/public representatives from these other backgrounds to help explain and promote the trial and even be featured in the PIS and videos.

Changes during the trial

The following may occur in studies that run for several years:

- Eligibility criteria are revised to exclude certain participants because of a safety concern.
- The control (comparator) therapy is no longer used in routine practice, and so needs to change.
- The event rate for the primary endpoint is much lower than expected (hence, the trial could be underpowered), so it is either revised or replaced with an alternative endpoint to yield more events. Alternatively, the recruitment target is increased, or follow-up is extended to yield more events using the original endpoint.
- The primary endpoint is superseded by a better endpoint.

Any of these key changes should be reviewed independently by a data monitoring committee (see page 187), or expert panel established just for this purpose. Changes to the trial protocol or other key procedures that may affect participant safety, scientific validity, trial conduct, or quality of the trial interventions are referred to as a **substantial amendment** that usually needs to be approved by the research ethics committee (and regulatory agency if applicable) before being implemented. Sponsors can implement **urgent safety measures** (USM) if there is an immediate significant risk to the health and safety of trial participants. This can be done without first seeking approval from the regulatory agency or ethics committee, though these organisations need to be informed in writing, with clear justification, usually within 3–5 days.

Statistical analysis plan (SAP)

The statistician drafts an outline of the statistical analyses to be performed at the end of the trial. This should include how each of efficacy, adherence, QoL and safety are to be analysed, including specific statistical methods, subgroup analyses and sensitivity analyses for dealing with multiple major endpoints, missing data or repeated measures. It should be finalised before the database is ready for the full analysis. The SAP would be included with submissions to regulatory and HTA agencies for licensing and market access.

Patients who decide to withdraw from the trial

Participants have a right to withdraw from a trial, but they can be asked why in case there is an emerging issue. It is essential to distinguish someone who withdraws from trial-specific procedures (e.g. clinic visits, blood tests) from another who withdraws consent for access to and use of all of their data and biospecimens (and hence outcomes). Investigators should always aim to continuously collect outcome data from medical records where possible, and most participants do not mind this. It is also worth requesting that all data and biospecimens collected up to the point of withdrawing can be used for the trial analyses and future research projects.

10.8 Monitoring the trial and suspension/early stopping

The level of monitoring necessary for each study depends on its complexity, potential risks to participants, and ensuring good scientific validity of the trial.

Protocol deviations can be reported by site staff or identified by the sponsor, such as:

- a participant was not strictly eligible according to the inclusion criteria (**protocol waiver**)
- an important health assessment/scan/blood test was missed
- a drug dose was lower or higher than it should have been.

Deviations can be minor. Major deviations could have a significant negative impact on safety or trial integrity (e.g. completeness or accuracy of major endpoints) and could be called **protocol violations**. Protocol waivers for eligibility are discouraged, but if they do occur, they need to be clinically justified and signed off by the chief investigator. Waivers can be avoided by using more flexible wording of the eligibility criteria, but without allowing recruitment of people who are not appropriate for the trial.

Protocol deviations or violations or other events where procedures have not been followed can be considered to be a **serious breach** if a participant is possibly/likely to be harmed as a result, which should be reported to the regulatory agency and ethics boards.

On-site monitoring involves a member of the trial team visiting a site, and checking medical records and other documents to confirm that participants really exist, that signed consent has been obtained, that data have been recorded correctly onto the case report forms (CRFs), and that adverse event reporting has been appropriate and timely. Pharmaceutical companies undertake a high level of on-site monitoring because they consider that application for a drug license is less likely to be declined. **Source data verification (SDV)** involves checking some entries on the CRFs and database with the original data in medical records. This can be done for all participants (100% SDV) or a random proportion of them (e.g. 10% SDV). SDV can be an expensive activity, and there is uncertainty whether it noticeably changes the main trial results. SDV may be done when the data quality for a particular site is questionable.

Due to costs, non-commercial organisations limit on-site monitoring activities (e.g. checking signed consent and serious adverse events have been reported on time). Central monitoring, using the electronic database can be done by the sponsor without visiting sites. This applies statistical methods to the database to identify errors on key variables, potential under-reporting of adverse events, or potential over- or under-dosing of trial drugs; any of which may trigger on-site monitoring. Central statistical monitoring is cheaper and easier to perform than full on-site monitoring and SDV.[5, 6]

Safety monitoring and reporting

Monitoring and reporting adverse events (AEs) is an essential function (called **pharmacovigilance** in trials of drugs or medical devices). An AE can be symptomatic or asymptomatic, and the different definitions are shown in Figure 10.4. AEs normally do not include progression or death when they are a natural consequence of the disorder of interest.[#]

SAEs should be reported to the sponsor (or coordinating centre) within 24 hours of discovery. SUSARs require special processing, and national regulatory agencies can have specific rules on how to classify an AE as a SUSAR. Fatal or life-threatening SUSARs

---

[#] But if an excess of disease-related deaths is seen this should still be considered 'harm' and acted upon accordingly.

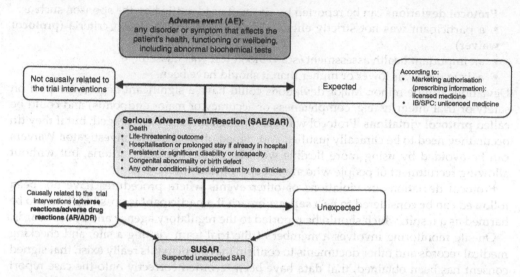

Figure 10.4 Adverse events. They can be judged to be causally related or not to the trial therapies; and expected or unexpected. A subset of AEs is called an SAE (defined above), and if it is serious and unexpected it becomes a SUSAR. IB, Investigator's Brochure; SPC, Summary of Product Characteristics.

must be reported to the regulatory agency by the sponsor, typically within 7 days of being notified by the site. If the SUSAR is not fatal or life-threatening, the regulatory agency is informed within 15 days. The REC or IRB that approved the trial protocol is also notified. The system and timelines are similar in many countries, including the EU, UK, US, Canada and Japan.

Expected AEs should be listed in the trial protocol because if serious events occur, they may not require expedited reporting (i.e. easier to handle). In the EU/UK, such expected events can also be listed in the Reference Safety Information (usually contained in the Investigators Brochure or Summary of Product Characteristics).

If unacceptable AEs are seen during the trial, an **urgent safety measure** (USM) can be implemented immediately, without prior approval by the regulatory agency (for trials of medicinal products); e.g. trial drug dose is lowered.

The sponsor submits Annual Safety Report to the regulatory authority, which includes:

• An analysis or summary of safety in the trial
• A list of all suspected SARs (expected or unexpected) to date
• A summary table of the suspected SARs.

Sponsors may also provide **24-hour medical cover**, where a clinician treating a participant can seek information about the trial and the treatments being evaluated. When an SAE occurs in a double-blind (placebo) trial, the treatment allocation may need to be revealed if considered necessary to treat the event (**emergency unblinding**). This can be done either via central trial staff or the electronic trial database, but the decision must be clearly justified. Unblinding is usually done for a SUSAR, though the trial clinician or trial staff at the site are often still kept blinded when possible.

Adverse events should be monitored in all trials by both site and central staff, especially for studies of medicinal products and devices. If they occur, the treatment could be modified accordingly if appropriate (e.g. dose reduction or delay, temporary discontinuation then restart after the event has resolved, or permanently stopped).

Ongoing independent review and monitoring

It is good practice that most trials have independent oversight to monitor their progress. This is done by an Independent Data Monitoring Committee (IDMC) or Data and Safety Monitoring Board (DSMB); a group of 3–5 health professionals and a statistician, with no direct connection to the trial. The composition, roles and responsibilities of the IDMC/ DSMB may be documented in a charter.[7] They regularly examine:

- adverse events, especially SAEs and SUSARs
- poor recruitment, and possible reasons for this
- data completeness, and whether there are lots of missing data from one or more sites
- issues about adherence to the trial interventions and other background therapies
- primary and key secondary efficacy outcome measures.

The sponsor submits a report to the IDMC/DSMB (typically every 6–12 months). Overly long reports (>100 pages) are unfortunately common. A shorter and focused report is preferable, and if anything major is found, the members can ask for more details. The report and review meeting can be in two parts: **open report** (IDMC/DSMB members plus trial staff and chief investigator) to examine accrual, data completeness and general issues, and **closed report** (panel members and the trial statistician only) to review efficacy and safety by trial arm.[#] For double-blind trials, the panel members could ask for the trial arms to be unblinded (in strict confidence). An IDMC/DSMB confidential review of interim efficacy data might avoid the need to pre-specify several formal interim analyses in the protocol, which increases the sample size.

The IDMC/DSMB can recommend changes to the trial protocol or PIS (e.g. change eligibility criteria), change the delivery of the therapies if there are unacceptable harms, or suspend or terminate the study early.

Suspending trials or closing them early

There may be several reasons why a trial must be temporarily stopped or closed early (Box 10.8). The decision is usually made and agreed by the trial team and the IDMC/ DSMB. Systems need to be introduced to inform sites and the participants already recruited (especially if there is a new risk of harm or the person needs to stop the trial treatment). The ethics committee, which originally approved the trial, should review and approve this information before it is sent to participants. Stopping guidelines can be pre-specified in the protocol (e.g. Table 4.2, page 50).

Interim efficacy analyses

Interim efficacy analyses are often done before a trial finishes recruitment and need to be handled with care.[8,9] These can be part of the design and sample size (e.g. **group sequential trials,** Section 5.10, page 72), otherwise deciding to stop a trial early is done when there is clear evidence of superiority or futility (Box 10.8). Stopping early should involve looking at several efficacy endpoints and perhaps key subgroup analyses, and the safety profile.

If stopping early for superiority (the new therapy appears beneficial), large early effects could be 'too good to be true'. In a trial comparing cardiovascular death between candesartan and placebo, the interim March 2000 analysis had HR 0.63 and $p=0.0007$.[10]

[#] Pharmaceutical companies usually employ an external statistician (through a contract research organisation) to do this.

Box 10.8 Reasons for stopping a trial early

- The objectives are no longer of interest, making the trial out of date.
- New information makes recruitment to one or more trial arms unethical or unacceptable.
- Poor accrual or the event rate is so low that the targets would never be reached.
- AEs with the new therapy are more common/severe and unacceptable.
- None of the primary or key secondary efficacy outcome measures show benefit (**futility**).
- Primary outcome shows a clear benefit that is highly statistically significant (**superiority**).
- Primary outcome clearly exceeds the non-inferiority margin (non-inferiority trial): the experimental intervention is less effective than the control group.

But the final analysis in 2003 had HR 0.91 and $p=0.055$. This example reflects 'regression to the truth' by completing the trial.

If stopping early for futility (the new therapy appears to not be beneficial), sufficiently reliable data are needed to avoid terminating a trial when the new treatment really is effective but takes time to show this.

Superiority: have a **stopping guideline**, where each interim analysis must achieve certain pre-specified p-value thresholds as evidence for early stopping (e.g. for first interim, second interim and final analysis, the p-values to define statistical significance could be $p < 0.0005$, $p < 0.014$ and $p < 0.045$[#] respectively).[8] Alternatively, use $p < 0.001$ at all interim analyses (Peto–Haybittle rule). The stringent earlier p-values ensure that there are sufficient participants/events.[10]

Futility: various methods exist, some require adjustments to the sample size or p-value at the final analysis, but use of **conditional power** does not. Box 10.9 illustrates the concept of conditional power. Generally, if it is ≤15% this might be low enough to conclude futility. But if the analysis is too early (e.g. <50% of the events have occurred), the futility assessment might be unreliable and the trial could be stopped early in error.[11]

10.9 End of trial

Several activities occur when a trial is due to end; Figure 10.5. The formal end of a trial (i.e. the point at which data collection will stop) may not be obvious. It could be after a defined period (e.g., 3 years after the last patient has been recruited), or after a certain number of events has been seen. The definition has implications for funding and study sites. The sponsor is usually required to notify the ethics committee when this occurs (e.g. within 90 days in the EU for IMP trials). Once the key data have been received and entered, the database is downloaded for statistical analysis, called **database lock** and this can occur several times afterwards for future analyses.

[#] It is not 5% because some of the overall 5% error rate has been 'used up' at early analyses, called alpha (a) spending. In the Peto–Haybittle rule, very little of the 5% has been spent early on, so the final p-value can still be compared against 0.05.

Box 10.9 Illustration of using conditional power to stop a trial early for futility

Targets for end of trial: number of patients 500, number of events 150, and hazard ratio 0.70.

First interim analysis: 200 patients, 58 events and observed hazard ratio is 0.85.
Conditional power is 38%*: based on the current data, there is a 38% chance of seeing a hazard ratio of 0.70 (or more extreme) that is statistically significant if the trial continued to the end (*assuming* the true hazard ratio is 0.70). This is a fairly high probability, so the trial continues.

Second interim analysis: 350 patients, 102 events and observed hazard ratio is 0.97.
Conditional power is 2%*: based on the current data, there is only a 2% chance of seeing a hazard ratio of 0.70 (or more extreme) that is statistically significant if the trial continued. This is a very low probability ($\leq$15%), so we might stop the trial early. But it is best to have a confirmatory interim analysis afterwards.

Conditional power is influenced by whether we have seen enough events yet. This is quantified by the 'information fraction'. For the first analysis, this is 39% (58/150 events), which is fairly acceptable. But for the second analysis, it is 68% (102/150), which is more reliable.

*There are formulae to calculate this for any type of effect size.

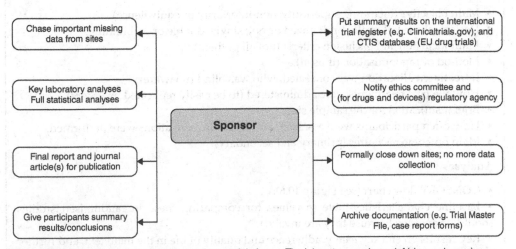

Figure 10.5 Typical activities undertaken when a trial closes. The laboratory analyses (of biospecimens) may help with interpreting the clinical results, including the identification of predictive biomarkers. These need to be pre-planned so that the main clinical trial report is not delayed.

The Trial Master File and the trial database should be kept by the sponsor for several years after the trial has closed, and recruiting sites also need to keep relevant trial documentation and participant CRFs.

It is also good practice to inform participants (if they are still alive) of the main results and conclusions; and this can be done via their clinician/health professional or the sponsor's website.

 Data sharing (including biospecimens and imaging scans) is a key part of collaborative research, and maximises the use and value of clinical trials. Data-sharing agreements (Box 10.6) need to be in place when the collaborator is external to the sponsor. Sending fully anonymised data (no personal identifiers such as names, date of birth, address, and the original trial ID number) usually has less restrictions than sending data with personal identifiers.

10.10 Reporting and publishing trials

All trials should be reported publicly, usually in a health professional journal, regardless of the findings, and this is a legal requirement in several countries for drug trials. There are established reporting guidelines for journals called consolidated standards of reporting trials (CONSORT).[12–18] Box 10.10 outlines the main sections and Figure 10.6 is a flow chart.

Box 10.10 Main items that should be covered in a typical clinical trial report/journal article

• Concise background and justification, including a statement on current disease burden/impact.

Methods

• Main objective (including superiority, non-inferiority or equivalence).
• Design: phase I, II or III; randomized or not; single, double or no blinding.
• Main inclusion and exclusion criteria (not all of them).
• Method of randomisation (if used).
• If treatment allocation was concealed, who was blind (unaware).
• How the trial treatments were administered (to be easily replicated by others).
• Brief justification for the sample size.
• How often participants were assessed, and which investigations were performed.
• Main outcome measures (primary and secondary).

Analyses

• CONSORT flow chart (see Figure 10.6).
• Baseline characteristics table (p-values for comparing these in randomised studies should be avoided because they are invalid).[19]
• Key results on efficacy, safety, adherence and quality of life in the main text; and further details in the online appendix.

Discussion and conclusions

• How the trial fits in with other evidence (e.g. other similar studies).
• Main trial design or conduct limitations.
• What information the trial has provided, and how it can be used (what happens next).
• Implications for participants, future research/trials, or understanding biological mechanisms of the new treatment.
• Conflict of interest statements for authors (e.g. personal financial or professional gain directly linked to the trial, or may be perceived to represent a potential bias).

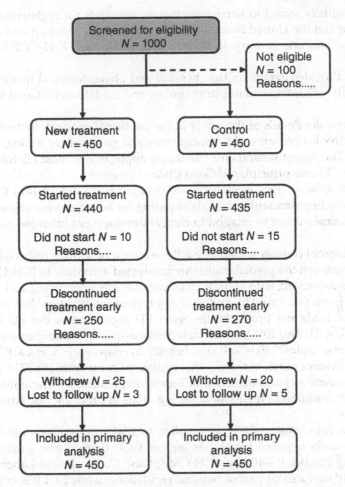

Figure 10.6 Outline of a typical CONSORT flow diagram showing recruitment and what happens thereafter.

10.11 Regulations and guidance associated with conducting trials

Clinical trials are experiments on humans. Those who participate are given an intervention that they would not normally receive, and they often undergo additional clinical assessments and tests, including having to complete questionnaires. It is therefore essential that their safety, well-being and rights are protected. This is the main purpose of the regulations and guidelines. They also ensure that the clinical trial data are valid and robust, and can be used to reliably demonstrate that the benefits of the intervention outweigh the possible risks.

The Declaration of Helsinki, developed by the World Medical Association (1964), represents ethical principles associated with conducting medical research studies of humans.[20]

Many clinical trial protocols and journal articles state that the study has followed the Declaration of Helsinki. These principles were later used to form the International Conference on Harmonization (ICH) guidelines for Good Clinical Practice (ICH-GCP); see Box 10.11.[21]

ICH-GCP initially aimed to harmonise the requirements for registering medicines in Europe, Japan and the United States. It is internationally recognised and allows clinical trial evidence from one country to be accepted by another. ICH-GCP has four major categories:

Q. Quality: Provides details on the chemical and pharmaceutical quality of the drug, such as stability, validation and impurity testing, and guidelines for Good Manufacturing Practice.

S. Safety: Provides details of the safety of the medicinal product, including toxicology and reproductive toxicology, and carcinogenicity and genotoxicity testing.

E. Efficacy: The largest section and one that is applicable to most clinical trials. It provides details of 13 core principles of Good Clinical Practice.

M. Multi-disciplinary: This section covers issues that do not fit into the other three categories, including standardised medical coding for adverse event reporting, and timing for pre-clinical studies in relation to clinical development intended to support drug registration.

Many commercial companies seeking a licence for a new drug (especially in multiple countries) ensure that the pivotal trial(s) are conducted according to ICH-GCP.

Regulations associated with clinical trials vary between countries, and they typically cover several items that apply to studies of any type of intervention; Box 10.12.

For trials of medicinal products, the main EU regulation is the EU Clinical Trials Regulation (EU-CTR 536/2014), which includes its own GCP guidelines, and is applicable to all EU member states.[22] EU-GCP significantly overlaps with ICH-GCP but has fewer requirements in some parts. In the US, the regulations come from the FDA (e.g. the Food, Drug, and Cosmetic Act and the Code of Federal Regulations).[23] There may also be specific regulatory attention to high-risk areas, e.g. trials in pregnancy or advanced cell and gene therapies.

The general principles of GCP are applied to trial interventions other than drugs, but are not usually required legally. As well as GCP, there is also guidance for Good Manufacturing Practice (GMP; e.g. ICH-GMP)[24] and Good Clinical Laboratory Practice (GCLP).[25] GMP may also be part of national regulations, while GCLP is largely guidance that aims to improve the quality and standards of translational research. Trials that include biospecimens to define eligibility criteria or primary biological endpoints, or as exploratory translational research, may follow GCLP guidelines, to ensure the validity and reliability of the laboratory techniques, assays and reagents. Box 10.11 outlines the key features of GMP and GCLP.

Box 10.12 National regulations tend to cover the following areas in relation to all clinical trials

Informed consent	Independent ethics review required	Storage and use of human tissue*
Data protection and confidentiality	Special groups (e.g. limited mental capacity, vulnerable adults, children and adolescents); and informed consent	Trials of medicines only: Good Clinical Practice Drug manufacturing

*E.g. blood, urine, normal or diseased tissue, skin, bone.

Box 10.11 Main features of Good Clinical Practice, Good Manufacturing Practice and Good Clinical Laboratory Practice

Good Clinical Practice (GCP)	Good Manufacturing Practice (GMP)	Good Clinical Laboratory Practice (GCLP)
Covers participants' rights, trial justification, and scientific robustness	*Sets out how trial medicinal products should be produced*	*Sets out how laboratories handle and test biospecimens from trial participants, particularly tests for key study endpoints*
• Informed consent must be given	• Manufacturing facilities and equipment must be constructed appropriately	• Facilities must be fit for purpose, with reliable systems and equipment for sample storage and analyses
• The potential risks of participating in a trial should be outweighed by the possible benefits	• Written SOPs should specify and validate the production processes	• Written SOPs should specify how samples are received, processed, stored and analysed
• The rights, safety and well-being of patients should prevail over the interests of science and society	• Processes to minimise/avoid contamination are required	• Each analytical method (assays, techniques) should be validated and fit for purpose
• Research should be conducted by suitably quali-fied health professionals		• Reagents should be suitably labelled, including storage instructions, stability and expiry date
• There should be prior research from preclinical (animal) studies		• A secure computer system should be used to record all details of samples from receipt, through analyses to destruction
• The design should be scientifically sound		
• Data should be kept confidential and protected		
• Systems should be in place to assure the quality of the trial conduct and quality and accuracy of the data		• Staff should be appropriately trained and qualified, and kept safe
• Independent ethics approval is required		• Regular audit and quality control are required

Data protection and confidentiality are key issues. Collecting personal data should be justified and approved by the ethics committee, and the participant should give specific consent. Several countries have national regulations that govern the collection, handling and sharing of personal data (e.g. the General Data Protection Regulation (GDPR) in the EU), with financial penalties for data breaches.

Audit and inspection (trials of medicinal products and some medical devices)

The regulatory agencies in many countries may inspect the offices of the sponsor, the trial coordinating centre, one or more study sites, the drug manufacturing facilities, or a laboratory responsible for biomarker testing particularly if the marker is integral to the design. These inspections can be pre-planned or triggered by an unexpected and urgent serious concern. A visit may last 3–5 days. The inspectors check that:

- all necessary regulatory and ethics approvals and signed agreements have been obtained
- all trial documentation (e.g., the TMF) is available, complete and up to date and insurance policies are in place
- GCP and GMP guidelines are followed
- there are clear systems for monitoring safety, and SAEs and SUSARs are reported on time.

Inspectors can suspend or stop a trial if they find serious issues, especially any that compromise patient safety.

Insurance and indemnity

Trial sponsors should provide insurance for non-negligent harm (physical or emotional injury or death) caused by participating in the trial, but where the protocol was followed correctly by site staff; e.g. a serious adverse event. This allows affected individuals to receive financial compensation from the sponsor's insurers (the sponsor would indemnify the recruiting site against such claims, i.e. the site would be protected). This insurance is different from that in a hospital, which has responsibility for the standard of care for a patient. If hospital staff have been negligent, for example, they gave the wrong trial drug or dose, compensation should be met by the insurers of their employer (for negligent harm), and not the trial sponsor (the site would indemnify the sponsor against such claims, i.e. the sponsor would be protected).

10.12 Why trials 'fail'

A 'failed trial' or 'negative trial' are commonly used terms when the primary effect size in a superiority trial is not statistically significant (p-value ≥ 0.05);[#] or in a non-inferiority study the effect size 95%CI includes the unacceptable non-inferiority margin.[26] But these

---

[#] But see section on the misinterpretation of p-values, page 94. Also, if a major secondary endpoint is statistically and clinically significant, focus might switch to this, but decision-makers would consider the appropriateness of this.

terms are misleading. They imply that the trial generated no new information and perhaps even wasted resources. In fact, all trials provide something useful, even if they tell us that a new therapy that was initially thought to be effective was truly not more effective than current standards of care. This means that future research and resources can focus on something else, or an investigation of the data and biomarkers could lead to new biological insights that lead to new research or a better designed (e.g. targeted) therapy.

The perception of a 'failed' trial contributes to publication bias (i.e. researchers are less likely to submit to journals, and some journals are less likely to review or accept for publication). Perhaps a better term is that the trial 'did not meet its objectives', but what is more important is to understand why. Investigators need to think carefully about how the study was designed, conducted or analysed, and whether any component could have led to the observed results. Box 10.13 lists reasons that investigators could consider, and some might be mitigated by design or conduct.

Before investigators firmly conclude that they have a 'failed' study, they should look at subgroup analyses (but with care), other efficacy endpoints, different methods of statistical analyses, per-protocol analyses, and consistency with other studies of the same intervention.

Box 10.13 Possible reasons why a trial does not achieve its primary objectives ('failed'/'negative')

- Recruited participants were not as expected or unrepresentative of the target population (e.g. higher or lower prognoses/risk).
- Poor accrual: lack of interest from sites, or participants were unwilling to enrol because they do not like the protocol (e.g. the trial therapies, or too many extra clinic visits/assessments).
- Event rate (e.g. number of cardiovascular disease events) is too low: trial is underpowered and inconclusive.
- The new intervention was inadequate, e.g. dose too low, treatment duration too short.
- Too many people on the control therapy crossed over to the new therapy, so the effect size shows a small or no effect (avoided by not allowing it in the protocol).
- Target effect size was over-estimated, so the trial was underpowered for a more realistic but smaller effect (i.e. p-value for the observed effect is just above 0.05).
- Primary outcome measure was insensitive or inappropriate to show a treatment effect.
- Many participants stopped trial treatment early (e.g. adverse events), hence unable to get the full benefit.
- Recent evidence makes the objectives obsolete/irrelevant, so the trial would be out of date when published.
- The control (comparator) treatment is no longer current standard clinical practice, or it has improved over time so the difference in efficacy between the control and new treatment is smaller than initially estimated.
- The outcome measure includes unvalidated biomarkers (e.g. insensitive or does not measure what it is intended to measure).

Checking the sample size assumptions

Checking the sample size assumptions with the observed outcomes might also indicate an issue with the trial participants and can be especially useful if a trial 'fails'. In the trial in Box 6.4 (page 89) the following checks can be made for the primary outcome measure:

| | Overall survival | | |
	Expected from the sample size (protocol)	Observed in the trial	Comments
Control group	Median 12 months	Median 14.3 months	If these are fairly similar (as they are here), it could mean that the trial participants were representative of the target population. If very dissimilar, the baseline factors might indicate the participants were too different from that expected and this might have affected the results.
Avelumab (experimental group)	Median 17.1 months	Median 21.4 months	This comparison might indicate if the new therapy has performed much better or worse than expected (here better).
Hazard ratio	0.70	0.69	This shows that regardless of the participants recruited, the target effect size was reached.

These checks are not infallible but if there are big differences in any of them, there should be a close inspection of, for example, the baseline characteristics, to see if any explain the differences.

References

1. Hackshaw AK. *How to Write a Grant Application: for Health Professionals and Life Sciences Researchers.* 1st edn, Wiley-Blackwell (BMJ Books), 2011.
2. Crocker JC, Ricci-Cabello I, Parker A *et al.* Impact of patient and public involvement on enrolment and retention in clinical trials: systematic review and meta-analysis. *BMJ* 2018; **363**:k4738.
3. Karlsson AW, Kragh-Sørensen A, Børgesen K *et al.* Roles, outcomes, and enablers within research partnerships: a rapid review of the literature on patient and public involvement and engagement in health research. *Res Involv Engagem* 2023; **9**(1):43.
4. Chan AW, Tetzlaff JM, Altman DG *et al.* SPIRIT 2013 statement: defining standard protocol items for clinical trials. *Ann Intern Med* 2013; **158**(3):200–207.
5. Kirkwood AA, Cox T, Hackshaw A. Application of methods for central statistical monitoring in clinical trials. *Clin Trials* 2013; **10**(5):783–806.
6. Buyse M, Trotta L, Saad ED, Sakamoto J. Central statistical monitoring of investigator-led clinical trials in oncology. *Int J Clin Oncol* 2020; **25**(7):1207–1214.
7. Damocles Study Group. A proposed charter for clinical trial data monitoring committees: helping them to do their job well. *Lancet* 2005; **365**:711–722.
8. O'Brien PC, Fleming TR. A multiple testing procedure for clinical trials. *Biometrics* 1979; **35**:549–556.
9. Pocock SJ. When to stop a clinical trial. *BMJ* 1992; **305**:235–240.
10. Pocock S, Wang D, Wilhelmsen L, Hennekens CH. The data monitoring experience in the Candesartan in Heart Failure Assessment of Reduction in Mortality and morbidity (CHARM) program. *Am Heart J* 2005; **149**(5):939–943.

11. Jitlal M, Khan I, Lee SM, Hackshaw A. Stopping clinical trials early for futility: retrospective analysis of several randomised clinical studies. *Br J Cancer* 2012; **107**(6):910–917.

12. https://www.equator-network.org/reporting-guidelines/consort/.

13. Butcher NJ, Monsour A, Mew EJ *et al*. Guidelines for reporting outcomes in trial reports: the CONSORT-outcomes 2022 extension. *JAMA* 2022; **328**(22):2252–2264.

14. Piaggio G, Elbourne DR, Pocock SJ *et al*.; CONSORT Group. Reporting of noninferiority and equivalence randomized trials: extension of the CONSORT 2010 statement. *JAMA* 2012; **308**(24):2594–2604.

15. Boutron I, Altman DG, Moher D *et al*.; CONSORT NPT Group. CONSORT statement for randomized trials of nonpharmacologic treatments: a 2017 update and a CONSORT extension for nonpharmacologic trial abstracts. *Ann Intern Med* 2017; **167**(1):40–47.

16. Calvert M, Blazeby J, Altman DG *et al*.; CONSORT PRO Group. Reporting of patient-reported outcomes in randomized trials: the CONSORT PRO extension. *JAMA* 2013; **309**(8):814–822.

17. Juszczak E, Altman DG, Hopewell S, Schulz K. Reporting of multi-arm parallel-group randomized trials: extension of the CONSORT 2010 statement. *JAMA* 2019; **321**(16):1610–1620.

18. Junqueira DR, Zorzela L, Golder S *et al*.; CONSORT Harms Group. CONSORT Harms 2022 statement, explanation, and elaboration: updated guideline for the reporting of harms in randomised trials. *BMJ* 2023; **381**:e073725.

19. Senn SJ. Testing for baseline balance in clinical trials. *Stat Med* 1994; **13**:1715–1726.

20. https://www.wma.net/policies-post/wma-declaration-of-helsinki-ethical-principles-for-medical-research-involving-human-subjects/.

21. https://www.ich.org/page/efficacy-guidelines.

22. https://health.ec.europa.eu/medicinal-products/clinical-trials/clinical-trials-regulation-eu-no-5362014_en.

23. FDA. Regulations: Good Clinical Practice and Clinical Trials https://www.fda.gov/science-research/clinical-trials-and-human-subject-protection/regulations-good-clinical-practice-and-clinical-trials.

24. ICH-GMP. https://www.ich.org/page/quality-guidelines.

25. Ezzelle J, Rodriguez-Chavez IR, Darden JM *et al*. Guidelines on good clinical laboratory practice: bridging operations between research and clinical research laboratories. *J Pharm Biomed Anal* 2008; **46**(1):18–29.

26. Pocock SJ, Stone GW. *The primary outcome fails – what next?* N Engl J Med 2016; **375**(9):861–870.

Clinical trial critical appraisal checklist

The checklist list below helps to focus on the main aspects of design, conduct and results. Some questions do not apply to all interventions and disorders. Most questions are phrased such that 'Yes' is a good thing (generally, the more 'Yes' responses the better). However, 'No' certainly does not mean it is necessarily a bad feature, and several 'No' responses do not necessarily make it a bad trial, but rather there is more careful consideration of potential bias and other impacts on the results.

Design and conduct features
1. Is this a phase I, II or III trial?
2. Is it a randomised study?
3. Is the experimental treatment (mode of delivery and access) appealing to participants?
4. Is the choice of control therapy appropriate/clinically relevant?
5. Was there any blinding (masking) of the interventions?
6. Was blinding necessary for this trial (why or why not)?
7. Is the delivery of the trial treatments the same between the arms (timing and duration)?
8. If the controls are allowed to crossover to the experimental arm, can this affect major endpoints?

Outcome measures
9. Are the primary and major outcomes clinically relevant?
10. Are they measured/ascertained/confirmed using standard/established methods?
11. Was an independent central review done? Was this necessary for this trial?

Size of trial
12. Is the target treatment effect reasonable and clinically worthwhile?

Follow-up
13. Is the follow-up schedule the same between the trial arms? If not, does this impact outcomes?
14. Were follow-up assessments frequent enough for the disorder and outcomes?
15. Was follow-up long enough for this trial?
16. Was loss to follow-up low?

A Concise Guide to Clinical Trials, Second Edition. Allan Hackshaw.
© 2024 John Wiley & Sons Ltd. Published 2024 by John Wiley & Sons Ltd.

Results

17. Did randomisation produce participant groups with similar characteristics?
18. Were the trial participants representative of the target patient group (generalisable)?
19. Was an intention-to-treat analysis performed? If not, why?

Efficacy

20. Was the observed efficacy result consistent with the target?
21. Was the expected effect in the control group consistent with that observed?
22. Interpret the main results: small, moderate or big clinical effect size, and relative and absolute effects. Consider reliability (narrow confidence intervals and small p-values). Consider consistency across different efficacy endpoints.
23. Was the treatment effect consistent across most/all subgroup factors? If not, consider whether there is strong enough evidence to make a definitive subgroup claim.

Adverse events

24. Which adverse events were more or less common in the experimental arm? Look at both relative and absolute effects because the latter might show less of an impact on participants.
25. Are the adverse events easy to treat (how serious are they)? Consider if they led to many participants who had treatment reductions/modifications.

Adherence and quality of life

26. Did a few participants stop trial treatment early?
27. Consider whether non-adherence was often due to adverse events (and what they were). Consider whether these events led to early stopping of the trial treatment for many participants.
28. Are the effects on quality of life clinically important? Do they actually matter to participants?

Overall interpretation, and put the trial in context

29. What is the overall assessment of the benefit-harm balance? Consider study quality based on the questions above.
30. What kind of analysis is in the paper: interim or final? If interim, what are the implications?
31. How does this trial fit in with other evidence (e.g. similar interventions for similar disorders; similar interventions for other disorders)?

Glossary of abbreviations used in clinical trials

AE	Adverse Event
ARR	Absolute Risk Reduction
ATMP	Advanced Therapy Medicinal Product
AUC	Area Under the Curve
BfArM	Federal Institute for Drugs and Medical Devices (Germany)
BICR	Blinded Independent Central Review
BSC	Best Supportive Care
CADTH	Canadian Agency for Drugs and Technologies in Health
CDSCO	Central Drugs Standard Control Organisation (India)
CHMP	Committee for Medicinal Products for Human Use (EU)
CI	Confidence Interval
CONSORT	Consolidated Standards of Reporting Trials
CRF	Case Report Form
CRM	Continual Reassessment Method
CRO	Contract Research Organisation
CTA	Clinical Trial Authorisation or Clinical Trial Application
CTIS	Clinical Trial Information System
CVD	Cardiovascular Death
DCGI	Drugs Controller General of India
DFS	Disease-Free Survival
DLT	Dose Limiting Toxicity
DSA	Data Sharing Agreement
DSMB	Data and Safety Monitoring Board
DSUR	Development Safety Update Report (EU/UK)
EFS	Event Free Survival
EHR	Electronic Health Records
EMA	European Medicines Agency
eTMF	electronic Trial Master File
EU-CTR	EU-Clinical Trial Regulation
EUnetHTA	European Network of Health Technology Assessment
FDA	Food and Drug Administration (US)
FWER	Family Wise Error Rate
G-BA	Gemeinsamer Bundesausschuss (Germany)
GCLP	Good Clinical Laboratory Practice
GCP	Good Clinical Practice

A Concise Guide to Clinical Trials, Second Edition. Allan Hackshaw.
© 2024 John Wiley & Sons Ltd. Published 2024 by John Wiley & Sons Ltd.

GDPR	General Data Protection Regulation
GMP	Good Manufacturing Practice
HR	Hazard Ratio
HTA	Health Technology Assessment
IB	Investigator's Brochure
ICER	Incremental Cost-Effectiveness Ratio
ICH-GCP	International Conference on Harmonization Good Clinical Practice
IDE	Individual Device Exemption
IDMC	Independent Data Monitoring Committee
IMP	Investigational Medicinal Product
IMPD	Investigational Medicinal Product Dossier
IND	Investigational New Drug
IQWiG	Institute for Quality and Efficiency in Healthcare (Germany)
IP	Intellectual Property
IPTW	Inverse Probability of Treatment Weighting
IRB	Institutional Review Board
ISRCTN	International Standard Randomized Controlled Trial Number
ITT	Intention-To-Treat analysis
JCA	Joint Clinical Assessment (EU health technology assessment)
LOCF	Last Observation Carried Forward
MACE	Major Adverse Cardiac Event
MAD	Maximum Administered Dose
MAIC	Matching Adjusted Indirect Comparison
MAMS	Multi-Arms Multi-Stage design
MED	Minimum Effective Dose
MHLW	Ministry of Health, Labour and Welfare (Japan)
MHRA	Medicines and Healthcare products Regulatory Agency (UK)
MTA	Material Transfer Agreement
MTD	Maximum Tolerated Dose
NCA	National Competent Authority (EU)
NHSA	National Healthcare Security Administration (China)
NICE	National Institute for Health and Care Excellence (England)
NMPA	National Medical Products Administration (China)
NNT	Number Needed to Treat
NNH	Number Needed to Harm
P&R	Pricing and Reimbursement
PBAC	Pharmaceutical Benefits Advisory Committee (Australia)
PFS	Progression-Free Survival
PD	Pharmacodynamics
PICO	Participants (Population), Intervention, Control/Comparator and Outcomes
PIP	Paediatric Investigation Plan
PIS	Patient/Participant Information Sheet
PK	Pharmacokinetics
PMDA	Pharmaceuticals and Medical Devices Agency (Japan)
PPIE	Patient and Public Involvement and Engagement
PROM	Patient Reported Outcome Measure
PSM	Propensity Score Matching
PSP	Paediatric Study Plan

PSUR	Periodic Safety Update Report
QALY	Quality Adjusted Life Year
QoL	Quality of Life (health-related)
QP	Qualified Person (EU/UK)
OR	Odds Ratio
OS	Overall Survival
RCT	Randomised Controlled (Clinical) Trial
REC	Research Ethics Committee
RMST	Restricted Mean Survival Time
ROC	Receiver Operator Characteristic curve
RR	Relative Risk or Risk Ratio
RWD	Real-World Data
RWE	Real-World Evidence
SAE	Serious Adverse Event
SAP	Statistical Analysis Plan
SDV	Source Data Verification
SE	Standard Error
SOP	Standard Operating Procedures
SPC	Summary of Product Characteristics
SUSAR	Serious Unexpected Serious Adverse Reaction
TGA	Therapeutic Goods Administration (Australia)
TMF	Trial Master File
TMG	Trial Management Group
TSC	Trial Steering Committee
TTF	Time to Treatment Failure
TTNT	Time To Next Treatment
USM	Urgent Safety Measure

Further reading

1. Griffin JP, O'Grady J (Eds). *The Textbook of Pharmaceutical Medicine*. 5th edn. BMJ Books, Blackwell Publishing, 2006.
2. Guyatt G, Rennie D, Meade M, Cook D. *Users' Guides to the Medical Literature: A Manual for Evidence-Based Clinical Practice*. 2nd edn. McGraw-Hill Medical, 2008.
3. Fiore LD, Lavori PW. Integrating randomized comparative effectiveness research with patient care. N Engl J Med 2016; **374**(22): 2152–2158.
4. Ford I, Norrie J. Pragmatic trials. N Engl J Med 2016; **375**(5): 454–463.
5. Pfeffer MA, McMurray JJ. Lessons in uncertainty and humility – clinical trials involving hypertension. N Engl J Med 2016; **375**(18): 1756–1766.
6. DeMets DL, Ellenberg SS. Data monitoring committees – expect the unexpected. N Engl J Med 2016; **375**(14): 1365–1371.
7. Yusuf S, Wittes J. Interpreting geographic variations in results of randomized, controlled trials. N Engl J Med 2016; **375**(23): 2263–2271.
8. Bhatt DL, Mehta C. Adaptive designs for clinical trials. N Engl J Med 2016; **375**(1): 65–74.
9. Pocock SJ, Stone GW. The primary outcome fails – what next? N Engl J Med 2016; **375**(9): 861–70.
10. Pocock SJ, Stone GW. The primary outcome is positive – is that good enough? N Engl J Med 2016; **375**(10): 971–979.
11. Mauri L, D'Agostino RB Sr. Challenges in the design and interpretation of noninferiority trials. N Engl J Med 2017; **377**(14): 1357–1367.
12. Woodcock J, LaVange LM. Master protocols to study multiple therapies, multiple diseases, or both. N Engl J Med 2017; **377**(1): 62–70.
13. Rosenblatt M. The large pharmaceutical company perspective. N Engl J Med 2017; **376**(1):52–60.
14. Moscicki RA, Tandon PK. Drug-development challenges for small biopharmaceutical companies. N Engl J Med 2017; **376**(5): 469–474.
15. Newhouse JP, Normand ST. Health policy trials. N Engl J Med 2017; **376**(22): 2160–2167.
16. Choudhry NK. Randomized, controlled trials in health insurance systems. N Engl J Med 2017; **377**(10): 957–964.
17. Frieden TR. Evidence for health decision making – beyond randomized, controlled trials. N Engl J Med 2017; **377**(5): 465–475.
18. Faris O, Shuren J. An FDA viewpoint on unique considerations for medical-device clinical trials. N Engl J Med 2017; **376**(14): 1350–1357.
19. Grady C, Cummings SR, Rowbotham MC, McConnell MV, Ashley EA, Kang G. Informed consent. N Engl J Med 2017; **376**(9): 856–867.
20. Pocock SJ, McMurray JJ, Collier TJ. Making sense of statistics in clinical trial reports: part 1 of a 4-part series on statistics for clinical trials. J Am Coll Cardiol 2015; **66**(22): 2536–2549.
21. Pocock SJ, McMurray JJV, Collier TJ. Statistical controversies in reporting of clinical trials: part 2 of a 4-part series on statistics for clinical trials. J Am Coll Cardiol 2015; **66**(23): 2648–2662.
22. Pocock SJ, Clayton TC, Stone GW. Design of major randomized trials: part 3 of a 4-part series on statistics for clinical trials. J Am Coll Cardiol 2015; **66**(24): 2757–2766.
23. Pocock SJ, Clayton TC, Stone GW. Challenging issues in clinical trial design: part 4 of a 4-part series on statistics for clinical trials. J Am Coll Cardiol 2015; **66**(25):2886–2898.

A Concise Guide to Clinical Trials, Second Edition. Allan Hackshaw.
© 2024 John Wiley & Sons Ltd. Published 2024 by John Wiley & Sons Ltd.

Index

Note: Page numbers in *italic* and **bold** refers to figures and tables, respectively.

A+B (e.g. 3+3) designs 33, 34, *34*
absolute effects 83, 91
absolute risk difference 81–83, **84**, *88*, *89*, 90–92, **97**, 100
accelerated titration design 34, *34*
adaptive designs 47, 60, 72
adherence 5, 16, 37, 55, 98–99, 136, 139, 159, 161, 187
adjusting *p*-values. *See* splitting *p*-values
advanced therapy medicinal products (ATMPs) 142–144
adverse events (AEs) 5, 15, 30, 37, 50, 79, 129, 159, 176
analysing 96–98
  monitoring 184–186
  reporting 55
  treatment-related 96
agreements (types of) 179–180
  data-sharing or material transfer 180
allocation bias 9
allocation concealment 9
alpha spending 188
analysis of covariance (ANCOVA) or of variance (ANOVA) 117
area under the curve (AUC)
  pharmacokinetics (phase I trials) *31*, 37
  prognostic markers 122, *122*
artificial intelligence 2
audit 194
audit trail (database) 176

basket trials 47, *47*
Bayesian methods/statistics 33, 43, 47, 96, 120
  indirect comparisons 155, 157–158
behavioural/lifestyle interventions 139–141
bias 4–5, 9, 11–12, 67, 69, 103, **109**, 135, 160
  allocation 9
  follow-up 12

publication 195
  selection 9
  withdrawal 12
bioavailability, pharmacokinetics (phase I trials) 31
bioequivalence trials 59
biological and targeted therapies 1
biomarkers 12–13, 16–17, 32, 44
  biomarker-driven phase II trials 47
  developing 124
  integration (in the design) 62, *63*
  predictive/prognostic 120–123
biospecimens 12, 17, 32, 62, 63, 170, 173, 175, 182, 184, 190, 192
'black box' warnings 130
blinded independent central review (BICR) 67
blinding. *See* placebo
Bonferroni correction 74, 114, 117–118
Bryant and Day phase II design 43

carryover effect 59, 115
case report forms (CRFs) 11, *172*, 175–176
  data collection and completion 181
  on-site monitoring 185
  types 175
cause-specific survival 24
categorial data/measures 18–19
cell therapy, *See* advanced therapy medicinal products
censoring 22, 88–89, 96
centile plot 21
central monitoring 185
chief investigator 170, 187
chimeric antigen receptor (CAR) T-cell therapy 142
clearance (CL), pharmacokinetics (phase I trials) 31
Clinical Trial Application (CTA) *172*, 178
Clinical Trial Information System (CTIS) 178
clinician/physician choice 64
cluster randomised trial 66, *66*, 117, 135
